ADVICE TO STUDENTS

Yoga Research Foundation
6111 S.W. 74th Avenue
South Miami, Florida 33143
Tel: (305) 666-2006

ISBN 0-934664-55-2

Library of Congress Catalog Card Number 91-066335

PRINTED IN THE UNITED STATES OF AMERICA

ADVICE TO STUDENTS

by
Swami Jyotirmayananda

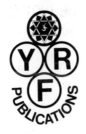

Dedicated
to those students
who aspire to attain
true success in their lives,
who will grow to be the ideal men and
women of tomorrow, paving the
way for peace and harmony
in the world.

PUBLISHER'S NOTE

In today's tense and highly complex world, students face great challenges. They must learn to use the technological tools of our society without allowing themselves to become over-mechanized and dehumanized. They must strive to fulfill their own desires for success and prosperity without becoming insensitive to the needs of others and the well-being of humanity.

Through his teachings, Swami Jyotirmayananda emphasizes the fact that if students do not give importance to the ethical and spiritual values of life, if they do not develop strength of character and follow the path of righteousness, then their education serves very little purpose. Although students may attain the highest academic honors, if they lack sensitivity to human and spiritual values of life and fail to develop compassion, generosity, and adaptability, then they will be unable to effectively shoulder their day-to-day responsibilities and enjoy harmony in their relationships with others.

Since 1985, Swami Jyotirmayananda has been bringing a new understanding of life to young people at the many youth retreats and Hindu conferences organized by the Vishwa Hindu Parishad and the local Hindu communities in Orlando, Atlanta, Boston, Pittsburgh and many other cities. The guidance Swamiji gave in these conferences and retreats was so appreciated that excerpts from these talks have been compiled into this present publication for the benefit of all.

This book offers unique insights into the important questions facing young people today as they strive to unfold their latent physical, mental and spiritual potential: how to develop willpower and self-reliance, how to concentrate the mind, how to enhance communication with one's parents and promote harmony at home, how to control fluctuating moods, how to become more physically fit, how to truly succeed in life. On every page, these questions and many others are answered with the depth of understanding, warmth, humor and wit that characterize Swamiji's profound, yet highly practical, teachings.

Advice to Students will prove to be a fountain source of inspiration to students of all ages who are seeking to know the secrets of self-improvement so that they can attain success and fulfillment in life. Filled with delightful stories and parables, this unusual book will become a constant companion to all those who seek joyous inspiration to meet the challenges of today's world.

We thank our staff for their devoted work leading to the printing and publication of this unique book.

May you attain success, harmony, peace, prosperity and Divine Enlightenment!

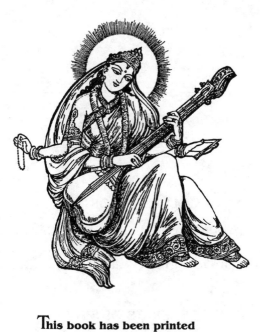

This book has been printed
to honor the following great souls,
whose family members (who wish to be anonymous)
have contributed towards the printing of this book
for the service of humanity:

Bhikhabhai Purshottamdass Patel (father) — Bandhaniwala
Chancelben Bhikhabhai Patel (mother)

Late Kanjibhai Patel (grandfather) — Kacchiawadiwala
Late Bhikhiben Kanjibhai Patel (grandmother)

Lalbhai Khushalbhai Patel (father) — Munsadwala
Sitaben Lalbhai Patel (mother)

Late Shri Radhey Shyamji Khandelwal (father) — Gwalior, M.P.
Shrimati Chameli Devi Khandelwal (mother)

Shri Narendra S. Shroff (father)
Late Shrimati Ila Narendra Shroff (mother) — Bangalore

**May God bless the donors
and their esteemed relatives — the above-mentioned
great souls — with His choicest blessings!**

CONTENTS

1
A GOLDEN OPPORTUNITY

Unfolding Your Potential 13
S-T-U-D-E-N-T 22
What Is Your Goal in Life? 35

2
THE SECRETS OF SUCCESS

What Is Success? 43
Thought Power 44
Willpower 47
Memory Power 51
Bring Order in Your Life 57
Be Self-Reliant 62
Repetition of Mantra 69
Prayer 72
Concentration and Meditation 79
What Is True Education? 90

3
UNFOLDING POSITIVE QUALITIES

A Divine Treasure Hunt 103
Who Is a Hero in the Battle of Life? 106
Ten Secrets for Living a Virtuous Life 108

The Joy of Sharing 144
The Importance of Good Manners 147
Vitamins and Minerals for Mental Health 153
Learn to Communicate Effectively 154

4
YOU AND YOUR FAMILY

Philosophical Insight into Family 159
Real Education Begins at Home 161
Give Reverence to Your Elders........................... 163
Honor Your Parents 165
The Value of Family Discipline 168
When the World Becomes Your Family 171
The Direct Path to Renunciation 173

5
FACING THE CHALLENGES OF TODAY'S WORLD

The Illusion of Sexual Freedom 179
What Is Brahmacharya? 182
Keep Your Spirits High!...................................... 188
Don't Fall Prey to Drugs! 192
Message to Hindu Students Living in the West ... 196

6
TOWARDS RADIANT HEALTH

Hatha Yoga Exercises 205
Pranayama Exercises 218
The Value of a Vegetarian Diet 224
The Search for Beauty 226
Enjoying the Gift of Sleep 231

Glossary of Sanskrit Terms 237

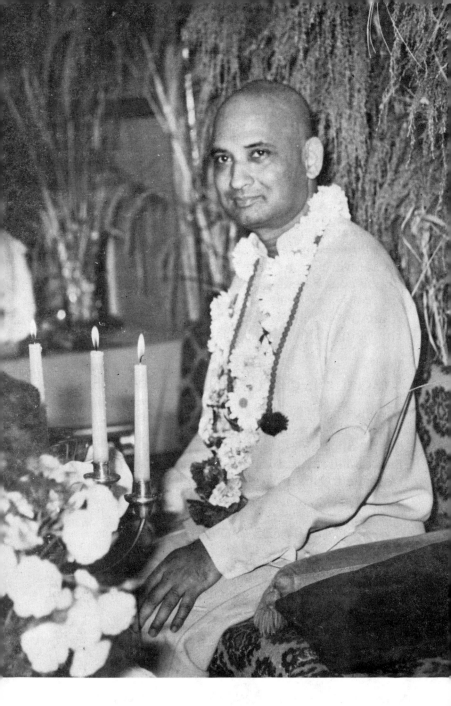

Author Swami Jyotirmayananda

1

A GOLDEN OPPORTUNITY

Live to
unfold your potential.
You have boundless resources
in the depths of your heart!

UNFOLDING YOUR POTENTIAL

Your student days are a golden opportunity for you to nurture all that is best in your personality. This is the stage of your life in which you lay down the foundation for your future. Therefore, you should make the most of every moment of this precious time. Apart from giving attention to secular studies, you must develop an inner sense of virtue that helps you to feel strong and confident about meeting the challenges of life.

Your education will not be complete unless you receive a "diploma" for developing the three great "H's": a heart that has compassion for your fellow man, a head that has creative thoughts, and hands that are dedicated to the service of humanity.

Keys to Success

Sincere effort joined with faith, perseverance, patience and understanding are the keys to success in every field of life. Study the stories of great saints and sages such as Krishna, Buddha, Jesus, Mahatma Gandhi, Swami Vivekananda, Ramakrishna Paramahamsa, Mira, Gargi, Madalasa, and other inspiring personalities from all over the world, and see how they behaved in the various conditions of their lives. Observe how faith, perseverance, courage, confidence, sincere endeavors and dedicated service have been the cause of their success and greatness.

Do not be the type of person who just sits and waits until opportunity arises. Instead, work hard to perfect yourself and move onward with firm determination day by day. As a result, you will have an abundance of opportunities that you never dreamed possible. There is a saying, "First deserve and then desire." But an even better principle is "Simply deserve, do not desire." When you are deserving, the Divine Plan automatically presents you with opportunities that are beyond all your expectations.

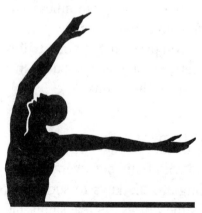

You Are the Architect of Your Destiny

According to yoga philosophy, everyone has boundless resources in the depths of his heart. By your self-effort you can undo the errors of your past and build a future of success and prosperity.

What you are today is the result of what you have been thinking and doing in your past. What you will be tomorrow will be the product of your thoughts and actions today. As you change your manner of thinking and acting, you can gradually bring about a change in your whole personality and mold a future according to your liking.

Never blame external factors for your bitter experiences in life. Assume responsibility for what you are and what you can be! Be bold and shape your future! Didn't men coming from the most adverse conditions rise to the highest levels of fame and glory through their self-effort?

Think Positively

There is no force in this world greater than thought, no power greater than thought-power. Therefore, think positively! By studying *The Art of Positive Thinking,* (see "Books" by Swami Jyotirmayananda at the end of this book), you can learn the art of developing thought-power. Elevate your thoughts by studying the *Gita*, the *Bible,* and other scriptures, as well as the yogic literature written by great sages and yogis of the world. By culturing your thought, you will shine as creative writers, poets, historians, philosophers, scientists and leaders of humanity.

Explore the Depths
of Your Mind

Your mind is like a huge iceberg. What you know of it is only a little tip of that iceberg. Beneath that tip lies a vast hidden area that needs to be explored, discovered, and utilized for your cultural and spiritual growth. One of the most effective techniques for exploring the hidden recesses of the mind is the practice of meditation. This practice begins with concentration of mind. When concentration becomes intense, it is called meditation. The following is a simple lesson for practising concentration:

Sit quietly in a cross-legged pose or in a chair. Close your eyes. Focus your mind on the center between the eyebrows. If the mind becomes distracted, bring it back again. Do not fight with the mind. Just watch its movements. Practise this for 15 minutes daily. In the beginning the mind will wander a lot in different directions and will not obey your directions. But after some time of repeated practice, it will behave like an obedient servant.

You may practise concentration on a variety of things. You may concentrate on an object such as a flower, or on a luminous flame, or on the picture of a Deity such as Krishna, Rama, Buddha, or Jesus, or upon anything else that your mind is attracted to.

You may also practise concentration by focusing your mind intensely on a small portion of material that you are reading for school or recreation. Read a paragraph and then close your eyes. Mentally visualize what you have read. Write it down from memory. Compare it with the original. By repeating this exercise often, your concentration and memory will greatly improve.

Concentration awakens your inner latent powers and enables you to have clarity of thinking and efficiency in action. You will be able to do a great many things in a short time if you have concentration of mind. You will radiate joy and cheerfulness around you. You will possess a magnetic personality.

Practise Asanas and Pranayamas

The scriptures say, *"Dharmartha kama mokshanam arogyamulam uttamam."*—Health is the foundation for the attainment of the four purposes of life, which are developing virtue, acquiring wealth, fulfilling desires, and attaining Liberation.

When you are physically healthy, your mind tends to entertain positive thoughts. "A sound mind in a sound body" has a great practical value.

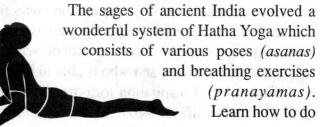

The sages of ancient India evolved a wonderful system of Hatha Yoga which consists of various poses *(asanas)* and breathing exercises *(pranayamas).* Learn how to do the headstand, shoulderstand, *Surya Namaskara* (twelve poses for adoring the sun), and the other important *asanas* and *pranayamas* that are explained in the last section of this book.

Make it a routine to practise these exercises for at least 20 minutes every day. This time will never be spent in vain. Rather, it will save you a lot of time in the future by preventing diseases, sickness and abnormalities of the body and mind. Be a yogi!

Discipline Your Speech

You are known by your words, so speak sweetly, but forcibly. If your words are lacking in force of character or strength of conviction, you will find it difficult to accomplish anything tangible.

Do not speak harshly or when you are overpowered by anger. If you do, you will repent later on. Be truthful, yet do not hurt the feelings of others when you speak.

Be a Real Hero in the Battle of Life

Who is a real hero? It is true that one who fights heroically in battle and defeats a big army is indeed a hero. However, one who is the master of his senses, his mind and his emotions, and who is able to become a fountain source of inspiration for others is a greater hero! One whose life flows out in service to humanity and in the promotion of peace and love is the real hero, the greatest hero. Be a hero!

In the light of yoga philosophy, you do not merely belong to one particular nation; you belong to the whole world. Recognize the One Self that indwells the hearts of all beings. You are that Self—not the physical body nor the limited personality.

Cultivate Virtues and Eradicate Vices

There are many positive qualities that should be cultivated in one's personality. Among these are non-violence, adaptability, charity, compassion, endurance, fortitude, humility, fearlessness, integrity, perseverance, self-control, contentment, purity, fearlessness, and devotion to God.

Contrary to these are the vices that should be eradicated: violence, anger, greed, lust, jealousy, arrogance, miserliness, insincerity, fear, discontent, fault-finding, smoking, indulgence in drugs, bad association, and any others that have a degrading effect on one's personality.

Developing a virtue is an art that you must learn with great patience. Suppose, for example, that you want to overcome pride and develop humility. You can accomplish this by reminding yourself again and again about the evils of pride, while, at the same time, reflecting upon the glorious advantages of humility. By studying the lives of great personalities such as

Mahatma Gandhi and others, you learn to deeply appreciate the power of their profound humility. Day by day, mentally assert, "I am growing in humility," and gradually you will develop that saintly quality.

Learn to detach yourself from whatever is negative within you, and continue to assert that you are growing in a positive direction. Keep a close watch over your mind, but do not become upset when a negative thought enters. Simply continue to direct your mind to the positive. Remember always that just as light removes darkness, virtue eradicates vice.

Study the Scriptures

It is important for you to study the scriptures of your religion and the religions of others. These scriptures abound with teachings that are intensely practical in resolving the problems of life. They hold the secret for peace and harmony within yourself and in the world around you.

Do not turn away from the scriptures by developing the notion that the stories contained in them are mere fairy tales. Far from this, the stories of the scriptures are highly mystical in nature. When you gain insight into their deeper meanings, you will be amazed at how much wisdom has been condensed in each and every story!

Young people of Hindu background would benefit greatly by learning Sanskrit or Hindi so that they may read the scriptures such as the *Gita, Ramayana, Mahabharata, Bhagavata* and the *Upanishads* in the richness of the language in which they were written. All young men and women of today, though growing up under the influence of a highly affluent and materialistic culture, should not forget their rich spiritual heritage—the spiritual wisdom that has been presented by the sages in the ancient scriptures and in modern commentaries upon these great works.

Live to unfold the potentialities of your soul. Practise the lofty ideals and the cultural values taught by the great teachers of mankind, and become a source of inspiration for others.

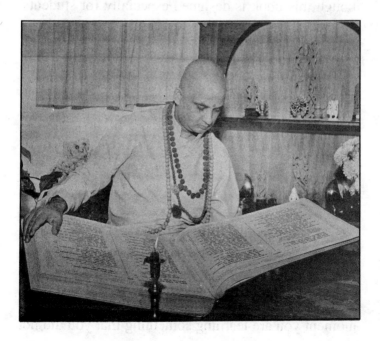

S-T-U-D-E-N-T

In the university of the world-process, everyone is a student. This broad understanding of the term "student" implies that one is continuously learning. Although this book is designed especially for students who are studying in schools and colleges, the following ideas apply to all human beings for the attainment of prosperity and success.

Since being a student is very demanding and time consuming, I have devised a simple method for remembering certain points which will help you to succeed in your studies as well as in life. All you have to do is simply think of the letters of the word "student": S-T-U-D-E-N-T.

"S" is for STUDY

Study has two aspects: academic study and the perpetual study of life. You are a student as long as you live, until you breathe your last breath. At every moment you are learning something that you did not know before. The eagerness to be open to learning must never stop. As Shakespeare wrote, "There are sermons in stones, and lessons in running brooks." And as the *Bhagavad Gita* teaches, "Every leaf of the cosmic tree is a *veda*—a source of knowledge."

In your academic studies, you must study systematically, regularly, and with self-effort. As a student, you cannot depend on anyone else. It is you who must study and learn; it is you who must prepare for examinations. It would be quite absurd to call a friend and ask him to do your assignments, saying, "Please study this history lesson for me. I'm too busy to do it!"

As a source of inspiration, reflect on the following story about the early years of an ancient saint:

There was once a boy who, prior to becoming a saint, was a very poor student. Because he had to work all day, the only time he was able to study was at night. Well one night he could not find sufficient oil to burn his lamp, so he went to bed in a state of frustration. When he finally fell asleep, an angel appeared in his dream and said, "I will give you all the knowledge in the world. All you have to do is open your mouth and I will spit the knowledge into it." The boy became upset and said, "No, please, that is not how I want to attain knowledge. I just want oil for my lamp so that I can study by myself and acquire knowledge with dignity."

Actually, the angel was just testing the poor student and because he was so pleased by the boy's response, he gave him blessings. Consequently, the boy became a great personality.

This story emphasizes the importance of depending only on yourself. With such a spirit of self-dependence, you too can become an excellent student as well as a great spiritual personality.

Believing in the power of your own self-effort, try to be organized in your studying. Before going to class, always try to prepare ahead for the next lecture. Glance through that subject and have an outline of the information. When you are prepared, your mind has a special capacity to attend to everything you hear. Otherwise, when you listen to a lecture for which you are not prepared, your mind goes blank. Consequently, you become upset and console yourself with the belief that "It's all right. Even though I don't have the faintest idea what is going on right now, I'll figure it all out when I get home."

Being a successful student is a great art, one that does not require you to have your head in books day and night. If you manage your time well, you can be prepared in an organized way. Therefore, it is not the quantity of time that you study, but the quality. So study well!

"T" is for TENACITY

Even though you may be weak in a certain subject, do not feel defeated—try again and again. If your effort is sustained with faith, you will succeed with the proper help and guidance. With tenacity, you can do amazing things. Nothing is impossible for anyone. So never for a moment accept the erroneous notion, "I am not meant for this!"

Suppose, for example, that you had to address your classmates by giving a short talk. You prepare your speech, but the moment you get to the podium you begin to tremble and your voice starts to waver. When you have finally gotten through it, someone tells you that you are not meant to speak publicly—"you don't have what it takes."

This is totally wrong. In the initial stage of all study, there is always a little wavering in your heart, a little diffidence. Yet everyone has the capacity to overcome this initial weakness. If you continue with tenacity, you will realize that every subject becomes interesting and engrossing—a form of exploration.

The idea that a project must go smoothly from beginning to end is wrong. No one becomes a hero in a battle unless he encounters some difficulty, some smack on the head! Therefore, tenacity must be adopted with great tenaciousness!

"U" is for UNDERSTANDING

The great secret of happiness lies in understanding, and understanding means many things. You must have a relaxed mind so that you can understand the academic subjects you are studying in school. You must understand other people, you must understand yourself, you must understand the meaning of the events in your life. As you become wiser and more patient, you must learn to avoid the misunderstandings that waste so much human time and energy.

As a simple illustration of such misunderstanding, reflect upon this story about a farmer and his ax:

There was once a farmer who was cutting wood with an ax. He had to go into his house for just a moment so he left his ax outside. When he came out again, he could not find the ax.

The farmer looked around and saw that a young man was walking near the house that was right across the way from his. He then thought to himself, "It must be him; he must have stolen my ax." The more the farmer looked at him, the more convinced he became that the young man was guilty. The farmer thought to himself, "Why, he not only looks like a thief, he even walks like a thief!" The more the farmer thought about it, the more agitated he became.

While he was getting all worked up, he suddenly turned around and, lo and behold, he saw the ax. In his rush to go into the house, he had apparently let it slip behind the door.

Once again he looked at the young man across the way. Only this time he thought to himself, "Surely he's a good person, for he not only looks like a good person, he even walks like a good person."

This humorous story reflects how quickly attitudes can change. When you misunderstand a situation, you interpret it in a faulty way. However, when you gain a correct understanding, you then interpret the situation in an entirely different way.

Understanding yourself and other human beings is a great art. It is much easier to be a student of botany or astronomy or grammar than to be a student of human nature. A human being is a most mysterious and profound being. Understanding human beings and relating to others in a harmonious way are challenges that continue day by day.

Understanding the meaning of life's events and developing a correct attitude toward adversity and prosperity are also vitally important challenges for every student of life. "Why," the mind asks, "should life present difficult situations before me?" Not finding the answer, it sinks in despair and depression and frustration.

However, if you tried to imagine what would happen to you if there were no difficult situations, if there were only prosperity, if everything happened according to your liking—you would realize that such a life would leave you like a spineless jellyfish!

To understand this better, look at a rosebush. Just as the thorns are absolutely necessary for the existence of this wonderful flower so, too, adversity is absolutely needed in your life. Just as each thorn allows the sap of the plant to be contained and evaporation to be controlled so, too, each adversity allows the "sap" of your inner strength to be revealed and contained. As that

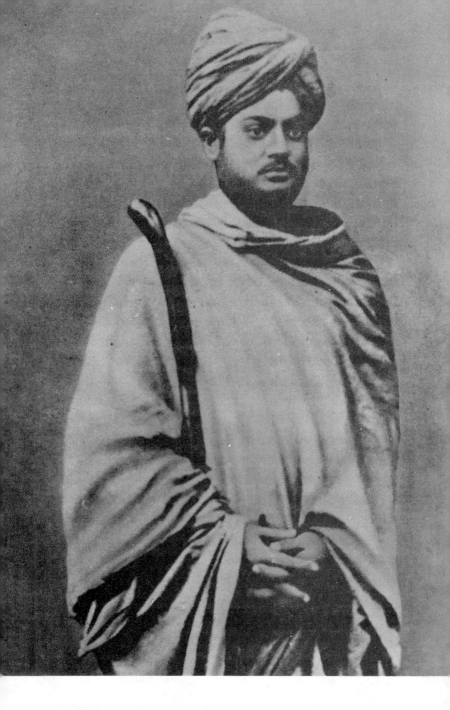

Sri Swami Vivekananda

"sap" accumulates, it eventually unfolds all the beautiful roses—the sublime Divine qualities—of your personality.

Remembering the importance of having proper understanding will lead you to a philosophical insight into yoga as well. The entire study of yoga philosophy is a matter of promoting understanding: understanding yourself, understanding the world, understanding your relationship to everyone and everything around you.

"D" is for DEVOTION

In the *Upanishads* there is a message given to students which states, *"Matri devo bhava"*—"Let your mother be your God;" *"Pitri devo bhava"*—"Let your father be your God;" *"Acharya devo bhava"*—"Let your teacher be your God." If we take this teaching one step further, we would assert, *"Deva devo bhava"*—"Let God be your God."

Although relating to God is your ultimate goal, you move towards Him in stages by developing Divine love towards those closest to you in family and society. First is your mother and your father. Apart from loving them in the basic human way, you develop the spiritual feeling that God is working through them.

In the Vedic culture, when a child first wakes up in the morning, he goes to his parents. He touches the feet of his mother and she blesses him; he touches the feet of his father and he blesses him. What is recognized in this act is that God is working through every individual. The child who is worshiping recognizes God in his mother and father. In turn, the parents recognize that it is God within them Who is blessing the child who is showing humility and reverence.

Developing the art of devotion begins at home. You love God by serving your elders, such as your mother, your father, your grandparents, etc. When you get older, you love God by serving your teachers.

Whenever you learn from a teacher, regardless of the subject, you should develop a special attitude of reverence and humility, so that his or her heart is in communion with yours. This deeper relation between teacher and student is the basis of receiving the highest form of education and culture. But from a more advanced point of view, "teacher" refers to a spiritual preceptor, or *guru*—one who guides you on that special path leading to Liberation.

Devotion must be nurtured little by little in your daily life through prayer, repetition of *mantra* (a sacred Divine name or a mystic formula such as Om, Rama, Krishna, or any sacred name according to your faith), and meditation upon the form of your Deity. There are different forms of worship in every religion, but love of God is the same. That love of God has to be developed by a student, for it is the basis for prosperity and higher attainment.

You may accumulate great wealth, fame, and power during your life, but if you do not have love of God flowing through your heart, life is meaningless. Some day you will age and you will no longer be able to enjoy the things you possess. Without devotion to God, you will face absolute despair and loneliness. But if you feel the Divine Presence within you, even when you age, even when death knocks at your door, your mind will be filled with peace and joy. Thus, devotion is the great treasure that makes all else meaningful.

"E" is for ERADICATION of Defects

Eradication of vices and cultivation of virtues will become possible if you develop the art of introspection. Do not waste your time looking for defects in others. Rather, look within yourself. Every evening, introspect by asking yourself if and how you went wrong: "Did I complete my assignments? Did I react unnecessarily in a certain situation? Did I say something to a friend or classmate that I shouldn't have?" It might even be a good idea to keep a diary and note what you did wrong; then, resolve to remedy the situation.

Never fill your mind with regret and sorrow over the defects you discover in your personality. Errors are natural in human development. A child must fall many times in order to learn how to walk upright. However, do not condone your errors either. Rather, face your errors with boldness! Eradicating vices and developing virtuous qualities must be constant and heroic projects throughout your life.

By introspecting, you will discover certain defects in your personality (like irritability, jealousy, anger, etc.) that tend to persist. There is an art to overcoming these defects; it does not require any form of deep psychoanalysis. Whether or not it is a result of the slap your mother gave you when you were four years old for breaking her favorite vase is not important. When and how you developed negative personality traits do not matter. What is important is that you learn the art of eradicating them.

You must gradually understand that deep down your spirit is full of love, that within you is the all-loving Self. Every day repeat to yourself the positive affirmation, "I am growing in love," and try to manifest that growing magnanimity of heart with the people around you. Think of sages and saints—how wonderful, loving, and kind they are. Then resolve to be like them and allow nothing to prevent you from attaining that goal.

By emphasizing positive traits, you cause the negative ones to gradually vanish. Even if they persist, it doesn't matter, because negativity does not have any substantiality. It is the positive that is your innate nature.

"N" is for NOW

Do not procrastinate. Do what has to be done now! Procrastination is the greatest obstacle to greatness and success. Great ideas may come to everyone, but the difference between the people who succeed and those who do not depends on how quickly they act on their ideas. Successful people put their ideas into practice. The people who don't succeed are the ones who say, "Oh, I have a great idea, but maybe tomorrow I'll have a better one. Actually, I'll wait until I have many good ideas. Meanwhile I'll store my ideas in the computer until I'm ready to take up the project perfectly, without one single flaw." Well, that will never happen!

If, on a daily basis, you work with your ideas and projects, handling your responsibilities and tasks as they arise, you will get everything done, and with much less pressure. On the other hand, if you postpone things for the next day, thinking that you will have more time then, other things inevitably come up. Then your tasks multiply, pressure builds up, and you get so frustrated that when you look at your cluttered desk you're tempted to throw everything away and do nothing.

When you attend to things as they come, your mind remains relaxed and uncluttered and your mental energy is free to be used for attaining internal fulfillment. However, when you are constantly pressured by time because you have not done what you should have done, there is no room within your cluttered mental space for peace and relaxation.

Therefore, remember, "D-I-N": Do it now! Never postpone until later what can be done now! Act on your good ideas now! Don't wait even one day!

"T" is for TARGET

One must always have a target, a goal towards which to strive. Professional and social goals should always be kept in view. Whatever you want to become, be it a successful scientist, a politician, or a religious person, strive to attain that goal. Never lose sight of the most important target—your spiritual target—Liberation. To be united with God is the ultimate goal of all studies.

Always remember with sincerity and determination what being a "S-T-U-D-E-N-T" implies:

S — STUDY
T — TENACITY
U — UNDERSTANDING
D — DEVOTION
E — ERADICATION OF DEFECTS
N — NOW
T — TARGET

If you remember this day by day, your experience as a student of life will be fulfilling and rewarding and you will attain all the goals you have set before you.

WHAT IS YOUR GOAL IN LIFE?

According to science, human possibilities are limited, but according to yoga philosophy they are not. According to yoga, you are a spirit, not the body; you are essentially the Self, not a limited personality. Therefore, you have within you unimaginable resources.

Science has not yet advanced sufficiently in the study of the mind to realize that there is no limit to your potentiality or to your success. These are limited only by the congestion of your own thinking, by the miserliness of your own view.

Think about all the truly great people that this world has known. What made each of them so great? All the elements that made these people great are in each of you. Each one of you could become like Mira, like Shankaracharya, like Mahatma Gandhi, or even like Buddha or Jesus.

You must decide what your goal is going to be in life, and then let that goal mold your personality. Once a student went to a spiritual teacher who asked him, "What will you do in your life? What is your goal?"

The student replied, "I want to pass my examinations, be well-educated, and get an impressive degree."

Then the sage asked him, "What are you going to do after you get your degree?"

"I will get a job, get married and have children."

Then the sage asked, "What will you do after that?"

"Well, I will educate the children."

"And what will you do after that?"

"I will grow old and the children will serve me."

"And what will you do after that?"

"I will grow still older and then I will die."

"Is that the goal of life—just to die?" said the sage. "There is a better goal—to try to understand your relationship with God."

God-realization is the true goal of life and true success means attaining God-realization. If you have attained God, you have attained all that is to be attained. There is nothing greater than that attainment.

As you move towards God, your personality blossoms and every good quality develops. You become a brilliant student and perform your duties in an excellent manner. You become a harmonious and relaxed person, bringing joy wherever you go.

With God-realization as your goal, you attain maximum quality in your life. But without God-realization as the goal, your life remains very shallow. You find yourself chasing one fleeting attainment after another, but never gaining real happiness.

Your mind may be overpowered by the desire to become rich. By the time you succeed in this, however, you realize how unhappy you really are and how many rich people there are around you who are also miserable. Then you think you would be truly happy if you gained skill in music or in some other art, and you work hard at this. Still you are not content. Restlessly, you chase one desire after another, looking in the wrong places for true happiness. Ultimately, however, complete fulfillment comes only when you are in tune with God within yourself.

The Horse with One Defect

In a humorous story from the Middle East, a man went to the market to buy a horse. While shopping around, he encountered an eager horse seller who declared, "My horse is the best; he has the most extraordinary qualities."

"Please tell me more about this unusual horse," the man said.

"My horse has such wonderful qualities. He is well built and extremely muscular. He has a long, silky mane, finely sculptured ears, beautifully enamelled teeth, and a powerful jaw. I could go on and on singing his praises."

"Well, is there anything that is not perfect in this horse?" asked the buyer.

"Yes," said the owner. "There is one defect."

"What is that defect?" replied the man.

"The horse is dead!"

Similarly, you may have money, fame, artistic talent, and popularity—but if you do not have the goal of attaining oneness with God within your heart, if you lack character and ethical values, you are just like the horse in the story: you have so many excellent things, but you are dead!

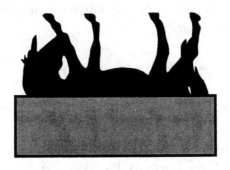

So Many Zeros!

A teacher in India with a good sense of humor used to give a mathematical illustration to show the value of love for God:

One zero equals only zero. But if you put one in front of that zero, you have 10.

Two zeros equal only zero. But if you put one in front of them, you have 100.

Three zeros equal only zero. But if you put one in front of them, you have 1000.

If you take the one away from 1000, what is left becomes zero.

Similarly, you may acquire so many things, but they are just so many zeros. But if you put love of God in your heart, that puts a One in front of all the zeros. In other words, with love of God in your heart, whatever you acquire becomes of value. Take God away from your heart, and your life becomes empty.

When problems develop in your life and other people do not seem to hear what you have to say, you must realize that God within you hears you. When you have to face difficult situations and no one comes to your help, there is a power in your heart that is going to help you. That power is God's power. Through God you can do amazing things.

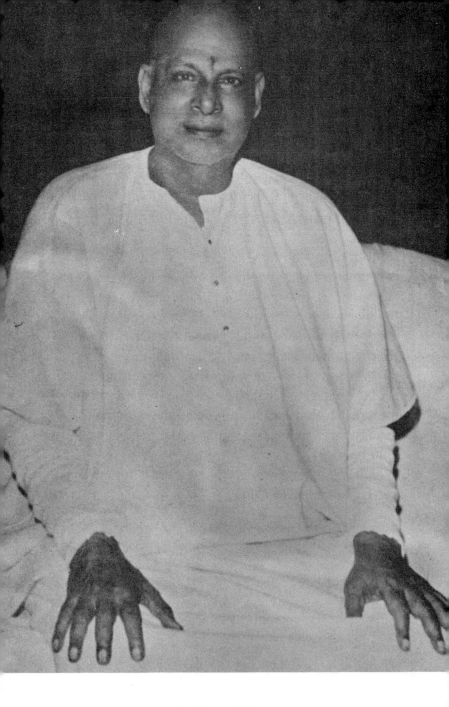
Sri Swami Sivananda

2

THE SECRETS OF SUCCESS

Assume
responsibility
for what you are
and what you can be.
Be bold and shape
your future!

WHAT IS SUCCESS?

Success has two aspects: relative success, or success in this practical world, and spiritual success. Although your ultimate goal in life is spiritual success, to reach that goal you must succeed in handling your practical realities with energy, skill, and imagination.

There is much more to success than being a high achiever in a field of study or doing well in business. To be truly successful is to be able to utilize the resources of your mind and to unfold the latent talents within you. If you are a truly successful person, you enjoy a sense of freedom and create a feeling of harmony and peace around you.

To attain true success, you must develop a balanced personality that is physically fit and mentally stable—a sound mind in a sound body! With mental stability as your foundation, you will be able to set the right goals for your life and make the self-effort necessary to attain success in the practical as well as in the spiritual realm.

THOUGHT-POWER

There is a wise saying that you should commit to memory and reflect upon often. If you carry its message in your heart always, you will be able to shape your thoughts as well as your future with dynamism and confidence:

> Sow a **thought** and reap an **action**.
> Sow an **action** and reap a **habit**.
> Sow a **habit** and reap a **trait**.
> Sow a **trait** and reap a **character**.
> Sow a **character** and reap a **destiny.**

By the tiny seeds of thought that enter your mind you are creating your future. There is a chain reaction that leads from what you think to what you experience as your destiny.

In the first link of the chain, a thought enters your mind and, on the basis of that thought, you act. For example, suppose you begin thinking, "I'd like to be more saintly, like Mahatma Gandhi or like Swami Vivekananda." In order to accomplish that desire, you set up a plan of action that will lead you in the right direction. You begin to organize your life so that your time is better utilized, and you vow to wake up earlier every day. Thus, on the basis of your thought, you begin to act in a different way.

For the first few days, waking up early is painful, and you feel sluggish. But if you persevere, waking up early eventually becomes your habit. Once that habit is formed, the day you oversleep you feel miserable. You become accustomed to waking up early and doing some exercises, some *puja* (worship), some prayer, some repetition of mantra (a divine name or mystic formula). Performing these practices in the quiet hours of the morning when nobody is around to distract you gives you mental relaxation and peace. When you begin to appreciate this, the repeated action has become your habit.

If a habit is sustained for a long time, it becomes a trait of your personality. Those traits can cause an overhauling of your entire personality and lead to a new definition of what people refer to as your character. That character leads you to the destiny or future that you experience.

With an understanding of this process, you find that you are the architect of your destiny. If you know the mystic art of shaping your thought power, you can become whatever you want to be.

For your thoughts to be effective in shaping your future, they must be clear and decisive. Once you have set a practical or spiritual goal, there should be no contradiction in your mind. Such internal contradiction reduces your thought power.

For example, suppose there are two boats that could take you across a river and you have to decide which one to enter. If, instead of wholeheartedly entering into one of the boats with both feet, you were to put one foot in one boat and the other foot in the other boat, neither of the boats would take you anywhere.

Similarly, in order to succeed in your practical and spiritual life, you must be decisive and clear thinking. Make a resolve about what you want to do and get on with it!

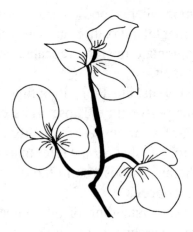

WILLPOWER

You have amazing power within that has not yet been tapped. Whatever you want, you can get. However, often what you want consciously is obstructed by your subconscious. Therefore, your will becomes weak and you don't get what you were after.

If you are weak-willed, although you may think of wonderful projects, you cannot succeed. You begin a new project or set a new goal for yourself, but then you forget all about it.

If you have willpower, you sustain your effort until you have accomplished what you set out to do. If you receive criticism or encounter obstacles, you are not discouraged.

Everyone wants to achieve great things—but those who succeed in doing so succeed because they had the will to sustain their efforts. That is the difference between one who is successful and one who is not.

The Man Who Wanted a Tattoo

There was a young man who suddenly developed the idea of having a lion tattooed on the muscles of his arm to make him feel more heroic. With that idea he went to a barber, who in olden days also did tattooing.

The young man said to the barber, "I am a lion among men! I want a lion tattooed on my arm!" "Very well," said the barber, and he began to prick the arm of the young man with his special needle and dye. Feeling that prick, the young man shrieked, "What are you doing to me?" The barber said, "I am making the paw of the majestic lion."

"Well, can't you make the lion without the paw?"

"All right," the barber said. "I will make just the face of the lion and not all the details."

So, the barber started pricking and again the young man shouted, "What are you doing now?" The barber said, "I am making the ear of the lion."

"Can't that lion be without the ear?" The barber said, "Well, all right, I have never seen a lion without an ear, but I will try."

Again he began pricking the young man with the needle, and again he cried, "What are you doing now?"

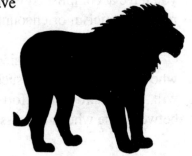

The barber said, "I am making the majestic mouth of the lion." The man said, "Let the lion be without the mouth!"

In disgust, the barber threw away his needle and said, "How can there be a lion without a tail, without paws, without ears, and without a mouth?"

Thus you see that the young man wanted to be lion-hearted and have a tattoo to prove it, but he couldn't stand the prick of the needle! You can't become a lion if you act like a mouse. If you want to attain greatness in life, then you have to endure some pricks in your life! Your will must be strong, despite all obstacles.

There is an interesting story that illustrates the power of patience and perseverance when all the odds seem to be against you:

The Conqueror and the Ant

Once there was a conqueror who was defeated in a certain battle again and again. Eventually, desperate and full of despair, he went into a mountain cave to commit suicide. As he sat there contemplating his death, he saw an ant climbing and falling, climbing and falling. The ant went on doing this seven times, until, on the eighth time, he climbed up the wall successfully. Seeing this, the conqueror said, "If I had as much patience as the ant, I could do it, too!" With renewed faith in himself, he tried again in battle and this time succeeded.

Like the ant, you must have patience and persistence. You have the Divine power within you, so if you persist you are going to succeed. Learn to wait and watch. Do not allow your will to become weak because of obstacles on your path. Things don't always turn out the way you expect them to, even though you have worked hard and tried your best. When that happens, do not become upset. Pray to God and continue doing your duties. With patience you will eventually succeed.

Willpower can be developed by simple exercises of self-discipline. If you have set a certain goal for yourself and you fail to accomplish it, discipline yourself in some intelligent way that will help to strengthen your will next time.

For example, if you have vowed to rise at 5:00 AM for meditation and you fail to do so due to laziness, then discipline yourself by skipping breakfast that day or by not taking any sweets. Or you can require yourself to study more of your school work on that day. If you discipline yourself in this way, you will develop willpower.

Or, suppose your words have hurt someone's feelings and you realize that you should not have spoken like that. Then practise *mauna,* or silence. Make a resolve that for two hours you will not talk to anyone. This will develop your willpower.

MEMORY-POWER

Having a keen memory is very important in your practical life as well as in your spiritual evolution. From a practical point of view, if your memory is weak, you will encounter difficulties not only in school, but in every aspect of your life.

If you truly understand what vast potentiality lies hidden in your mind, you will realize that you are capable of amazing powers of mental retention. You can unfold these powers and train your memory to serve you well by using the following techniques.

Develop Keen Attention

When you are inattentive, you frequently forget things. On the other hand, when you develop keen attention, you are always able to remember the things which are important in practical life.

Therefore, devote some time every day to focusing or concentrating the mind. If you do not do this, forgetfulness becomes normal. Concentration and meditation, *japa* (repetition of *mantra*) and *satsanga* (good association) are all effectively related to memory culture.

Remember What You Read

Try to increase your concentration when you read. You can accomplish this with the help of a simple exercise. Study a small passage from a book with an alert yet relaxed mind. Then close the book and try to see how much you can remember from that passage. Do this exercise again and again, and gradually you will develop greater memory power.

Learn to Associate Ideas

It becomes much easier to memorize things when you develop the technique of idea association. For example, suppose you have to remember a number like 539. It is helpful to build an association with each number. If you are philosophically orientated, you may associate the number 5 with the five elements. Similarly, the number 3 may remind you of various triads: there are three *gunas* or modes of nature; there is subject, object and their interaction; there is past, present, and future. The number nine is a number that possesses a unique mathematical constancy: no matter by what number you multiply it, the numbers in the product of that multiplication add up to 9. For example, 9x2=18 and 1+8=9; 9x4=36 and 3+6=9.

If you are required to remember various key points about one of your school subjects, you may try to come up with a symbolic letter that represents each point and then form those letters into a word you can easily remember. For example, in my grade school days we were once asked to memorize ten factors that determine the climatic conditions of a place. I still remember the acronym LANDS FORMS: L – latitude, A – altitude, N – nearness to the sea, D – direction of prevailing winds, S – soil, F – forest, O – ocean currents, R – rain, M – mountains, S – slope. In this way, all ten points were easily remembered.

In our ashram in Miami, Swami Lalitananda has composed a song entitled "Life Is a Delight." D refers to discipline, E to energy, L to reverence for life, I to integrity, G to God, H to harmony, and T to truth. Each time you sing about DELIGHT you remember so many valuable ideas for your spiritual life.

Focus on What Is Important

Different types of jobs require different types of memory skills. If you are a policeman you should remember how tall a person is, the color of his moustache, what type of glasses he wears, etc. If you are not a policeman, you do not have to torture your mind trying to remember such things.

Do not make your mind into a "garbage can" that holds all types of unnecessary memories; rather, your mind must be selective. Remember things that ought to be remembered; forget things that ought to be forgotten. Generally, people do the opposite: they remember things that are unnecessary and forget things that are important. As a result, their minds become cluttered and their lives are in turmoil.

When you are studying your school work, you must learn the art of going after the essentials, not the non-essentials. With good concentration, you can know immediately which points to focus on and how to organize those points so that your mind can grasp them and recall them in the future.

Handle Exams Skillfully

What is the difference between one who gets good grades on an exam and one who does not? Sometimes the difference is very little. Both may have memorized and understood the same things, but the student who gets the higher grade knows the art of test-taking.

When you have to answer questions on an examination, plan your time in such a way that you answer the questions you are sure of first, and do not sit brooding with tension over the ones that seem more difficult. As you answer the ones you know, you build up self-confidence and your mind relaxes. Then even the difficult questions may begin to seem more reasonable, and you realize that you remember more than you thought you did at the start.

Strengthen Your Will

Memory, will, and thought are related, just as fire, heat, and light are related. If you have strong will, you will be able to remember things well.

Never say to yourself, "Oh, I am a weak person." Always affirm the positive. Internally you are not weak. Your possibilities and your resources are endless. So make the affirmation, "My memory is improving and becoming stronger every day."

Discover Higher Forms of Memory

By adopting simple methods such as these, you can enhance the practical aspects of your memory. But a greater goal before you in life is to cultivate the kind of memory that helps you to learn meaningful lessons from the past. Such a memory shows you how to handle adversity wisely, how to make decisions thoughtfully, and how to develop your relationships with others harmoniously.

A healthy memory of this type enables you to recall an experience from the past without undue egoistic distortion or exaggeration. Such a memory is illumined by virtue and wisdom, and serves as a noble instrument for your spiritual evolution.

As you mature, you learn that it is a virtue to "forget" certain negative happenings in life. If someone has harmed you in some way, try, with a philosophical understanding, to forgive him. Face him with an open mind, not with a memory of his wrongdoing.

If you cannot do this, negative thoughts will start pouring into your mind like the monsoon rains. The resulting unhealthy memories will then create pain and poison your mind.

A healthy memory, on the other hand, causes positive memories to flourish. In that relaxed and happy mind, you will recollect mystical experiences of harmony, of inner fulfillment, of Divine Grace. This is

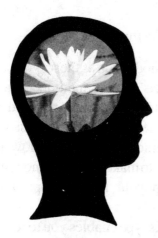

a highly advanced form of memory which elevates your personality and helps you to attain intuitional revelation of the Self.

Only in a relaxed mind can you recollect "I am *Brahman*—the Absolute Self, not this mortal personality." That revelation is the highest recollection possible. With that revelation, memory reaches its climax. With that remembrance, all fetters, all limitations are destroyed, and all *karmas* are annihilated. You become one with *Brahman*, or God—the Absolute Self.

BRING ORDER INTO YOUR LIFE

Make a Schedule

When you use your mental energy wisely, will-power increases. When you waste your mental energy, your will decreases. How do you waste your mental energy? By not having order in your life.

Suppose that today you wake up at 6:00, tomorrow at 8:00, and another day at 10:00. Suppose that today you go to bed at 8:00, tomorrow at 10:00 and another day at 12:00. With such a disorganized use of time, your willpower will become very weak.

Evolve a schedule in which the important things in your day can be done comfortably at a certain time. Do not make the schedule too strenuous. If making a schedule is difficult for you, seek help from someone who knows how to budget his time well.

Schedule your day from morning to evening so that everything is in balance. Allow time for play and entertainment, as well as for study and the performance of your duties.

Start Your Day Right

Try to develop the habit of getting up early; between 4:30 AM and 6:00 AM is fine—but don't sleep later than that. Once awake, use these serene morning hours to prepare yourself in a peaceful way for the day's activity.

Begin your day with prayer. Learn any prayer from the religious tradition of your family, or offer prayer to God in any way that comes naturally to you in your own words, according to your own personal feelings.

Learn to practise *japa* (repetition of *mantra* or any Divine name), a little concentration, and some yoga exercises. All this takes hardly any time at all and later it will save you the time and money required for visiting psychiatrists or going to hospitals. In all ways, these practices will save you from lots of troubles in your life.

After you have done your spiritual practices in the early morning, mentally make some resolves, such as, "Today I am not going to lose my temper. I will watch out for anger. I will develop patience." Armed with resolves such as these, start your day with confidence and inner peace.

Develop Good Study Habits

As much as possible, try to prepare ahead and be ready for the situations that you must face. Learn to be the master of every situation you encounter in school and in the world around you.

Every day look at your schedule of upcoming classes—geography, history, science, mathematics, literature, etc.—and try to prepare ahead for them. If your teacher is going to lecture tomorrow about a particular subject, try to read ahead about it in a general way—without going into too much detail—so that you'll have some idea of what you are going to hear.

If you do that regularly, your mind will develop a greater fascination for learning. When you already know something about what the teacher is saying, you become more alert and eager to learn.

When you enter a class feeling prepared, you are the master of the situation. Whatever the teacher says will seem like a feast for your ears. On the other hand, when you are not prepared, you dread everything, thinking, "This is a difficult topic. What if I can't learn it? What will happen to me if I fail?" Burdened with such negative thoughts, you feel like a slave of life, not its master.

Taking good notes during lectures is another important art. Certain things will impress your mind as being particularly important and interesting. Write them down so you can reflect upon them more deeply at a later time. Certain things may confuse you and will need further clarification. Write those down too so that you can ask your teacher more about them. Strive for quality, not quantity, in the taking of notes, and focus on only what is important. If you observe these points, you will find that keeping good notes can save you a lot of time and energy.

Value Time

Place great value on time at all times! Saving time and energy is very important if you want to succeed. For example, develop the habit of putting things in the right place. If you leave your possessions around in a haphazard way you are bound to loose a lot of time unnecessarily. A hundred times a day you will have to ask yourself questions such as, "Where is the book that I need for class? What happened to my watch? Where are my keys?"

Don't procrastinate! Try to do all your jobs promptly, and do not leave for tomorrow what you should do today.

There is one area, however, in which procrastination is encouraged: when you are very angry and you feel like doing something wrong that you will be sorry for later! When you angrily think, "Let me write a nasty letter to that person," tell yourself, "I will not write that letter today. I will write it tomorrow." By tomorrow your anger will probably cool down, and you will see things differently. As a result, you may completely lose interest in writing the letter and thus save yourself from much future trouble.

But in all good things there should be no procrastination. When a good idea comes into your mind, act upon it. Tomorrow will bring its own challenges and duties.

Be prompt! Never think, "Why should I arrive there on time? Everyone else will be coming half an hour late, so why shouldn't I also come late?" That is wrong. Be a person who has pride in principles. Adhere to time, even if others do not. By doing so, you help yourself and many other people.

Economize on labor! Evolve a life style that allows you to do maximum work in minimum time, with good precision and quality. As a student, you may have a great many tasks to accomplish for school as well as for your family. If you know the art of economizing on labor and utilizing time well, in a short time you will be able to do all the tasks in an excellent manner. If you do not know that art, it will take you a long time to finish your work, you will worry about everything constantly, and because 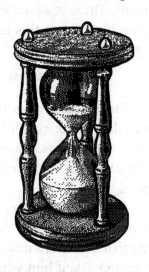 you are doing so many things in a distracted manner, the end result will not be as good as it could be.

BE SELF-RELIANT

For all those who seek happiness, peace and success in this world, self-reliance is the key to all attainments. There is a parable from the *Mahabharata* that gives insight into this great virtue:

The Farmer and the Fish Pond

There was once a farm in which water had collected, forming a shallow pond in the field. That little pool of water was linked to a bigger reservoir of water, and soon fish began to live and thrive in that shallow pond.

One day the farmer told the youngest of his three sons to go and empty that water from the field. When the fish overheard this, they went to their wise leader fish and asked him what they should do. The leader replied, "Do not worry. The farmer's son is very lazy. He will not do it. We have nothing to be concerned about."

The next day the farmer gave the same instruction to his second son, and the following day to the third son, but they both ignored it. Finally he said, "Tomorrow I am 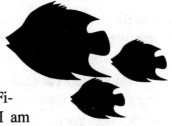 going to do it myself." The moment the leader fish heard this, he said, "Now we hear a warning sound! Let us flee from here to the bigger body of water. Since the farmer himself wants to do the work, it will get done!"

The idea conveyed by this parable is that when any project is done by yourself, without depending upon others, then you are at least ninety-percent secure that it will get done. When you depend upon others, however, you have no such sense of security.

How to Develop Self-Reliance

The art of self-reliance has to be developed from childhood. However, most children want to be lazy, to be dependent. That should not be so.

Do not become dependent upon others. Try to become more and more dependent upon yourself in both little and big things. This will give you a sense of great freedom later in life.

Don't depend upon your parents for bringing discipline into your life. Parents have their own problems. It is you who must live your life. Therefore, try to discipline yourself. Learn to get up early, to practise meditation, to do your duties at home without constantly being reminded, to set your own goals for your school work, etc.

Your parents are not your secretaries. Do not have them organize your desk, your room and your closets, while you go on shouting, "Mother, where is my pencil? Where is my pen? Where is that book? Where are my shoes?" Rather, know how to put things where they belong. If you know how to categorize things and put them in order, you save a lot of time.

You should know how to take care of your clothes and clean your room. When you are hungry, you should be able to prepare food for yourself. Learn a little bit about cooking from your mother, so that if she is sick, or if she is away, you can cook for yourself.

You should be your own servant, rather than have somebody serve you. Be proud of being able to do the things that have to be done, and of helping others rather than of being helped.

Don't develop a sickly image of success, thinking that it means having servants all around you so that you don't have to do anything. That is not success at all.

If there is a need to pull, you pull; if there is a need to lift bricks, you lift them; if there is a need to run, you run; if there is a need to carry something on your head, you carry it. That is success. Don't be fussy about little things. You can adapt to the needs of whatever situation you are placed in.

You should never have the idea, "Why should I act like a servant when my parents have enough money to employ servants?" People who adopt that philosophy of luxury do harm to themselves, because in spite of the external show of riches and luxury, internal diffidence and a sense of weakness develop within the mind.

In India, rich people generally become very dependent on servants because there are so many servants available to do even the smallest of tasks. Every little thing is done by somebody else. When a difficult situation arises when they are alone, they become like fish out of water. They do not know what to do. Even making tea can put one in a miserable predicament!

However, when you learn the art of self-reliance, you discipline yourself to do many things, not only for yourself, but for others as well. This allows you to discover that you have boundless resources, and that you can advance and rise to higher levels according to your determination and resolve.

A sharp distinction has to be made between depending on someone and being guided. In the development of self-reliance you should seek advice and allow yourself to be guided by those who are wiser than you. This guidance enables you to discover your own inner resources, and utilize them toward the attainment of Self-realization.

Self-reliance is an art that one must develop with great precision. It involves self-introspection, self-analysis, self-improvement, and self-discipline. All these qualities are inter-linked. When you learn that art you begin to develop confidence in yourself and your willpower becomes strong. You become aware that the source of inspiration and strength you are tapping is God within you, the Universal Self. Therefore, you have endless possibilities.

The King Who Learned Self-Reliance
From a Little Girl

Let me share with you another parable that provides insight into the great virtue of self-reliance. There was a king who listened to a priest reciting the entire *Bhagavata*, a scripture recounting the glory of Lord Krishna. At the end of every volume of that great work, there is a *'Mahatmya'* which means, "The benefit of this is that you will attain Enlightenment and become free of the world-process." The king, therefore, heard this promise of freedom again and again during the reciting of the great work.

After the entire reading of the *Bhagavata* was finished, the king asked the priest, "Have I become enlightened? Have I become liberated?" The priest replied, "You have to decide that for yourself."

The king said, "No, I have not attained Liberation. Therefore, what you are teaching is false. And for false teaching I will have you beheaded—unless you can give me a rational explanation of why I remain unenlightened."

The priest did not have a rational explanation to give. He didn't know what to say. So, feeling miserable, he went home. When his little seven-year-old daughter asked him why he was so sad, he informed her that the king wanted an explanation about why he had not attained Enlightenment after hearing the *Bhagavata* recited since that was the promise made again and again in the scripture.

The girl said, "It is simple. Take me to the royal court tomorrow and I will explain it to him."

So the next day the priest took his daughter to the royal court. When the king came and sat on the throne, the girl ran right in front of him and caught hold of one of the pillars of the palace, shouting, "This column has caught me; how can I be free, how can I be liberated?" The king said, "Let it go, you foolish girl, let it go!" But the girl kept on shouting and the king became angrier and angrier.

Finally, the girl said, "O king, aren't you doing the same thing? You are clinging to your ego, to your vanity, and unless you let go, you cannot be liberated. So why do you blame my father?" After hearing these words of wisdom, the king understood.

As this story points out, Enlightenment depends upon your own Self. You can study about it in the scriptures, and the guru can guide you, but ultimately you must work for your own Enlightenment. If you were to say, "I will tell my guru to pray for my Enlightenment, and his prayers will confer upon me

Liberation," you would be wrong. There is no harm in asking for prayer to help you attain Liberation, but you must understand that it is you who must work for it. If somebody could bring Enlightenment to you on a platter, he could also take it away from you. Enlightenment is something that you, yourself, achieve. If it is somebody else's achievement, it is not worth having.

Thus, strive to cultivate the virtue of self-reliance. It is by that virtue that you can integrate yourself, discipline yourself, attain success in every project, and finally attain Liberation. When you are self-reliant, you become dependent upon the big Self within you, and in that dependence lies absolute independence.

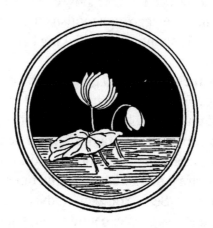

REPETITION OF MANTRA

Japa, or repetition of *mantra*, consists of repeating a mystic formula or Divine name many times. For example, you may repeat *Ram*, *Om*, Lord Jesus, or *Om Namah Shivayah* or any *mantra* that helps you to feel the Divine Presence within your heart.

Japa can be done with a *mala* (rosary) or without a *mala*. Receive a *mantra* from a spiritual teacher or choose one of your own. You can repeat it loudly, which is called *vaikhari*. You can repeat it semi-verbally, which is called *upanshu*. Or you can repeat it silently, mentally, which is called *manasik*.

Each time you repeat *mantra* you create positive impressions in your unconscious. You plant a seed of spiritual strength. Even if you do it mechanically, it still has its influence on your unconscious and will help you immensely in the future. Someday you will realize big changes in yourself.

That is why the scriptures speak so highly of *mantra*. Saint Mira said, "I found the wealth of the

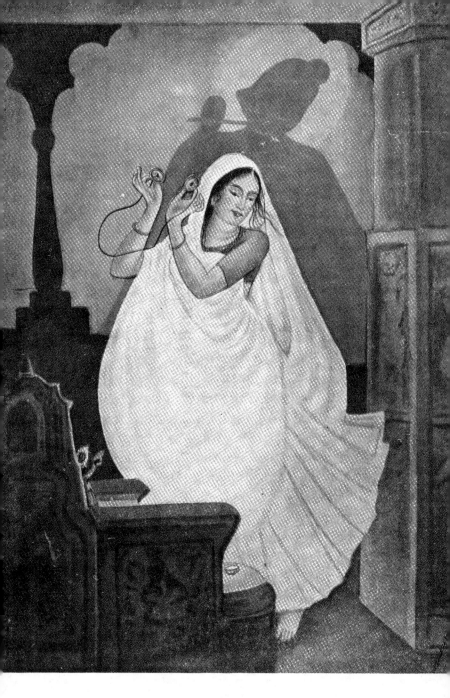

Mira — a woman saint of India
(Sixteenth Century)

Divine name—Rama. Other wealth decreases, but this wealth grows day by day and there is nothing like it." Tulsidas, Kabira, and other saints have also spoken highly of *mantra*. A simple *mantra* like *Rama, Rama, Rama* or *Om, Om, Om* will help you develop immense mental power.

By constant repetition of a Divine formula, the mind becomes charged with positive vibrations and, therefore, acquires the strength to withdraw itself into a state of concentration and meditation.

For students, one important *mantra* is that of Goddess Saraswati: *Om Sri Saraswatyai Namah*. While you repeat this *mantra*, allow your mind to think about the Goddess and meditate on Her presence.

Goddess Saraswati is the Goddess presiding over the intellect, over learning, over all talents. She rides on a swan, which is the symbol of a pure mind. The musical instrument in her hand, called a vina, symbolizes harmonization. When the strings are tuned correctly and are not too loose or tight, then beautiful melody flows. Similarly, the strings in your personality—reason, will, emotion, and action—must be harmonized.

While repeating the *mantra* of Goddess Saraswati, mentally feel Her presence—the presence of an all-loving Mother. By her grace all things can happen.

PRAYER

The Power of Prayer

Prayer is uplifting, inspiring, and fascinating for the mind and it has great power. Therefore, it is very important that each of you learns to pray. Through prayer you purify your mind and gain spiritual strength. Prayer is the foundation of success.

As you learn to pray, you must develop profound faith that your prayers are being heard. As a matter of fact, you can talk to God even more vividly than you can talk to other people around you.

When you talk to people, they do not listen completely because every human being is limited. God, however, can listen to you in the most profound manner because He is your innermost Self and knows all your thoughts. Even before you ask for something, God knows. You must understand that God is the dearest of all. He is more real than any person in the world. He is father, mother, guru—He is all.

Through your prayer you can help your parents and other grownups. When you are a child, you feel so small and they seem so big, and it seems that you cannot do anything for them. This is not so. In your mind you are big. In your heart you are big. So, if you learn the art of praying with a sincere heart, you can help the grownups immensely.

If you see your mother in difficulty and there is nothing you can do physically to help her, then sit down and pray to God. If you see your friend in difficulty, pray to God. Through the mighty force of prayer you can help even the most powerful people in the governments of the world handle their problems more effectively.

Developing love of God through prayer is the greatest attainment. All the studies in schools and universities won't give you anything equal to the joy of love of God. As you get older, you will not have to go to psychologists and psychoanalysts to solve your problems and ease your tensions. With love of God you will have very few problems.

Mahatma Gandhi offered prayers every day. But one day he missed his prayer, and he felt so miserable that he was trembling. Seeing this, one of his friends told him, "The very idea that you feel miserable about missing your prayer is, in itself, an act of tremendous virtue." To prove his point, the friend related a parable:

The Devil and the Saint

Once there was a saint in the Middle East who unwittingly remained sleeping when it came time for prayers. Seeing this, Satan came to his bedside and began to awaken him. The saint woke up and looked at Satan in surprise, saying, "How is it that you, who are well known for distracting people from prayer, are telling me to pray? Have you become a saint?"

The Devil replied, "Indeed not. But I know that if you do not pray now, later you will repent and that repentance will reach God's ears even more keenly than your prayer. Therefore, I can't let that happen!"

When Should You Pray?

Although you can pray to God at any time—while lying down, walking, or performing any action—it is good to also set aside time to pray when you can sit down quietly, with a concentrated mind, at a peaceful hour of the day. Early in the morning when you first awaken or before every meal is an excellent time to open your heart in prayer.

Praying just before you go to sleep is also highly effective. At that time, review the things that you did during the day and try to see what errors you have committed. Did you hurt somebody's feelings? Did you become angry? Did you speak lies? If so, pray to God for the strength to correct the errors.

What Should You Pray For?

When you pray you can ask for whatever you like, no matter how little or how great. For example, you may pray for the smallest things: "Let there be no mosquitoes in my room!" Or you may pray for success on an examination, or for a safe journey, or for good health.

You can pray for others as well as for yourself. When you ask for good things for others, that prayer carries a greater spiritual value than when you pray only for yourself. When you pray for others, your own well-being is automatically taken care of.

If your mind is mature, you will pray for strength and understanding in carrying the burdens of life. Do not ask God to lighten your load, but to give you strength— so that no matter what load you have on your head, you will be able to bear it lightly. If your strength increases, you can even hold an elephant on your head! But if your strength decreases, then even a butterfly becomes a terrible burden.

In the highest form of prayer,

you allow your feeling to flow towards God and ask only for more prayerfulness, more devotion, more awareness of Divine sweetness, more will to attain Self-realization.

No matter what you pray for, prayer is elevating for your mind. And prayer for even the smallest of things is better than no prayer at all.

How Should You Pray?

Prayer can be practised in many ways. You may use your own language when you pray, as if you are talking to God. When you pray in the language of your heart, try to develop a feeling of real closeness to God. This form of prayer will eventually lead you to an experience of internal silence in which no language is necessary at all to communicate what you feel.

A parable is told about a simple farmer in the congregation that was once led by Moses. This farmer could not understand all the sophisticated teachings given by Moses about a God without form, a God beyond all. So he decided to express his own inner feelings and pray in words he understood.

One day he sat down and said, "Oh God, I will wipe your face with my own handkerchief and I will stitch your clothes and I will find shoes for your feet...!" When the scholarly members of the congregation heard him use his own words in this way, they were very upset, for it seemed to them that he was acting against the high teachings and thus committing blasphemy. Even Moses himself was concerned, feeling that he could not allow that farmer, who was expressing what seemed to be a lower stage of prayerfulness, to remain in his prayer group.

But then one night Moses had a vision in which God appeared and told him: "That farmer is a greater devotee of Mine, though he is using simple words. Go beyond the words and look at his feeling. For him I am the only reality and all his sentiments are centered on Me—even though he is using ordinary language."

So, as the parable points out, you can use your own words in prayer, as long as your heart is open to God. It does not matter whether or not your words are grammatically correct or poetically arranged. All this does not matter. You may use whatever language comes to you.

Or you may use prayers that have been composed by great sages. While praying, you can bring to your mind certain passages from the great scriptures of your own religion or the religions of others. These religious scriptures are the source of all that is great in the whole world.

In the *Upanishads*, the *Bhagavad Gita*, the *Ramayana*, the old and new testaments of the *Bible*, and the *Quoran*, for example, there are numerous prayers that you can commit to memory. These prayers give you guidance about what to pray for, as well as insight into how to pray.

Make a hobby of writing down some beautiful prayers, keeping them in your pocket, and reflecting upon them again and again. That hobby will help you to explore the deeper resources within you.

Whatever form of prayer you adopt, what is important is that your prayer must proceed from your heart. It should be infused with profound feeling and immense sincerity. Such sincere prayer will lead you to the highest in life—to discover your internal relationship with God, to remember God spontaneously at every moment, and to live and move in God at all times.

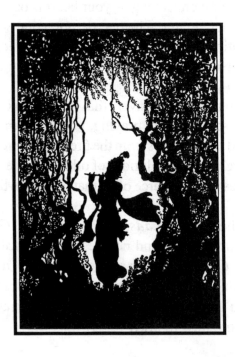

CONCENTRATION & MEDITATION

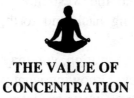

THE VALUE OF
CONCENTRATION

You can give a monkey a big title, make him the manager in charge of a million dollar business, put a hat on his head, and give him a necktie and a wonderful coat, but he cannot be really successful in that situation. So, too, it is with people. If you cannot control your mind, you are like the monkey. You may get great external power and wealth, but you remain internally restless like the monkey, and your prosperity will have no real meaning.

If you watch your mind, you will see that it is constantly jumping. However, if you could train it to stay on any one thing for ten minutes, you would experience the development of a special energy within you. This unique energy that results from concentration enhances your intellect, your emotional faculty, and your imaginative capacity. It awakens your latent inner powers and enables you to have clarity of thinking and efficiency in action.

If you develop concentration, you can do in two hours what would normally have taken you six hours to accomplish. When the mind is distracted you move in one direction at one moment and in another direction the next moment; you may move to the east five steps and then back to the west three steps. If you are constantly moving back and forth, nothing can be accomplished.

Without concentration, you may study a book for hours, without ever knowing what you were reading. If someone asks you what you just read on the previous page, you won't remember.

When you have concentration, as soon as you open the pages of a book you know how to identify the important points and organize those points so that your mind can grasp them. You know how to distinguish between the essentials and the non-essentials.

The Swan and the Crow

Once on an island there dwelt many crows who were very arrogant and thought that they were the most superior birds. One day a swan came to that island and the leader crow approached the swan, saying, "How many types of flights do you know?"

The swan said, "I know only one way of flying." "Well," said the crow, "I know 99 ways of flying and I challenge you to a race. Whoever reaches the first tiny island out there in the middle of the ocean will be the winner." The swan said, "I am not really interested in this race, but if you insist, let's go."

Both birds then started flying out over the ocean. The crow began to show off all the different flight patterns he knew. He went straight up, he went in a spiral, he flew at right angles, he made zigzag patterns. But in a short while he became exhausted and started sinking in the water.

The swan, who was flying forward with simple, graceful movements, looked back and saw the crow collapsing. Having compassion for the unfortunate bird, he swooped down and picked him up, balanced him on his back, and brought him back to the shore. When the crow had rested a bit, the wise swan said, "It is better to know one way of flying that can get you across than to know so many ways that get you nowhere."

When you are distracted, you are like the crow: you come up with so many projects but you do not fully succeed in any of them. But when you have concentration, you are like the swan and you will be successful in whatever you undertake. Whether you are trying to reach a practical goal in this world, or whether you are trying to advance spiritually towards the ultimate goal of Self-realization, if you have good concentration of mind, you will keep the goal clearly before you and move towards it in a meaningful and purposeful way.

INSTRUCTIONS FOR
CONCENTRATION AND MEDITATION

Set aside one room in your house or a separate part of one room for the practice of meditation. Keep that room as a shrine so that the moment you enter it, your mind will be filled with spiritual vibrations. You may choose to burn incense sticks before you start meditation.

Early in the morning, at the time of sunset, or in the evening before you go to bed are the best times for meditation. At these times the mind is calmer and more receptive. The atmosphere is serene and laden with spiritual vibrations.

Practise meditation for five minutes to start with. Then increase your time to ten or fifteen or thirty minutes each day.

Be very regular in your practice and do not be disheartened if you do not seem to be succeeding in the beginning. Every time you try to meditate, fresh grooves are being cut in your subconscious mind to replace the old grooves based on mental distraction. Eventually these grooves of meditation will allow you to enter into a meditative state without difficulty.

Try to maintain the serene and sublime feeling of meditation even during the active hours of your day. Let this feeling continue to flow on, like the silvery stream in the Himalayas.

EXERCISES IN CONCENTRATION AND MEDITATION

Meditation begins with concentration, or focusing on one idea so that the mind doesn't constantly jump around. As your mind becomes more and more still, your concentration automatically becomes meditation—the effortless and continuous flow of mind towards a single object or a central thought.

Concentrate on a Concrete Object

Practise concentration by putting a picture of Krishna or Rama or Jesus or any spiritual ideal before you, and place a lighted candle in front of the picture. Then gaze with eyes open at the candle flame and, through that flame, see the picture illumined.

Steady gazing with eyes open is called *tratak*. As you gaze, do not strain your eyes; close them whenever your eyes feel tired. Then open them again and continue to gaze at the candle flame. Each time you close your eyes, try to visualize the Divine form in the picture illumined by the light.

You may concentrate upon anything you like most—whatever you are drawn to, whatever is elevating and inspiring. You may concentrate on the shining moon, on a particular star in the night sky, on the rising sun, on the waves of the ocean, on distant mountains, on a beautiful flower, on a color or sound or other sense perception, or on any object of your choice.

Repeat this practice of concrete concentration again and again, day by day. It will relax your mind and help train it for more advanced methods of concentration and meditation.

Be a Witness to Your Mind

Sit quietly, close your eyes, focus your mind between the eyebrows and simply watch the movements of your mind. Do not fight with the mind if it jumps around like a monkey. Just watch its movements like a spectator, like a noninterfering witness. In the beginning, the mind will wander a lot in different directions and will not obey your directions or suggestions, but after some regular practice, your mind will behave like an obedient servant.

Concentrate on Abstract Qualities

If you concentrate your mind on the purity of Buddha, on the virtuous qualities of sages and saints, on the concepts of eternity and infinity, on the all-

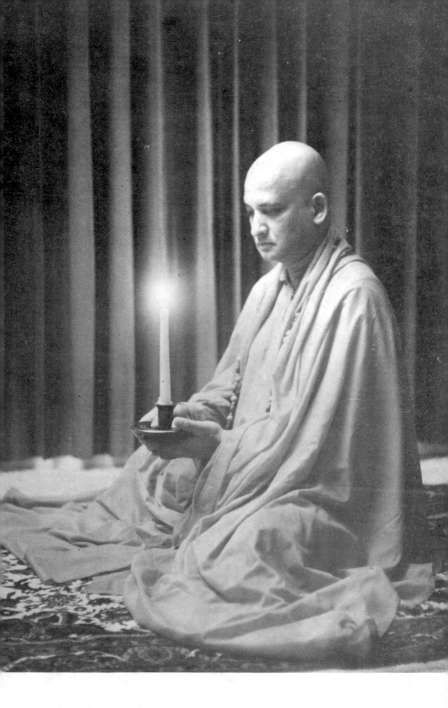

Sri Swami Jyotirmayananda

pervading presence of God, on peace, bliss or love, you are practising abstract meditation. Often this form of meditation adopts symbols for assisting the mind. For example, you may meditate upon purity as symbolized by the white snow on the mountains, or Divine radiance in the form of the brilliant sun, or infinity in the form of the vast sky, or the fullness of God in the form of the surging ocean.

You may meditate upon love by feeling that kindness and compassion flow from your heart like streams of rain flowing from the sky. Visualize your love permeating the entire universe as clouds of good wishes for all mankind emerge from your mind and shower within the hearts of all beings.

Meditate on Prana or Cosmic Energy

Visualize golden clouds of Divine energy entering into your *ajna chakra*, the mystic center between the eyebrows. Feel that your brain and nervous system are receiving the gentle rain of refreshing energy from them. Feel the waves of refreshing joy sweep over your body from the top of your head to the tips of your toes.

Meditate on the Mystic Ocean

Visualize a vast ocean before your eyes. Feel that you are sitting at the sandy shore watching the waves rolling onto the beach and then gracefully returning back. Listen to the heaving sound of the ocean as you watch the incoming and outgoing movement.

Next, let your vision expand to the waves that rise and fall. See only the waves on all sides. There is no shore, no sandy beach. You feel as if you are riding the waves. You feel as if you are being rocked by the arms of the ocean.

Enjoy the peacefulness of the moonlit night. The full moon is shining upon the waves, creating a shimmering, luminous path of light across the vast ocean.

Now dive into the ocean and go deep beyond the waves into the great silence of its profound depths. There are no waves, there is no moon; there is only profound peace and expansion.

After a while, allow your ego and your sense of individuality to melt in the vastness of the ocean. Feel that you have become the ocean, and your rolling waves are reflecting the light of the moon.

Meditate on Bliss

Feel that you are the Self, the ocean of Bliss. Different forms of happiness experienced by other people, by animals, by all living beings exist in the ocean of your innermost Self as waves and ripples. The joy that reflects in the morning breeze, the joy that awakens the buds to bloom, the joy that makes the deer dance in the forest, the joy that spurs nature to put on different attires of exquisite beauty—that joy is an expression of the ocean of the Self, the ocean of Bliss. That Self you are!

Meditate on Om

Place a picture of *Om* in front of you, and gaze steadily at that Divine symbol. Then chant *Om* as sweetly as you can for at least 5 minutes. Close your eyes after you finish chanting and just meditate on the sound of *Om* that lingers in your mind. Develop the awareness that *Om* is the absolute sound of the universe—it is the essence of all sounds everywhere in the world. It is part of You.

When you are seated outdoors in a peaceful spot, allow your mind to focus on different natural sounds around you, such as the humming of insects, the stirring of leaves in the wind, the singing of birds. Feel that all these sounds are emanations of the sound of *Om*.

Mentally repeat *Om* and let your mind develop an intense feeling of love towards the Supreme Self. Every mental utterance of *Om* should be like an eager step towards the Divinity.

As you continue to mentally chant *Om*, feel that you are touching the Supreme with every *Om*. Feel that the various Divine qualities—fearlessness, universal love, peace, bliss, wisdom, and dispassion—are flowing into your personality as an act of Divine grace.

Devotional Meditation

Seated at a little temple or shrine that you have created in your home, light a candle and place it in front of the picture of your deity—Rama, Krishna, Shiva, Jesus—or any other symbol of your Divine ideal. As you gaze at the candle and see the face of the Deity glowing behind the flame, allow your mind to relax. Think of nothing else but the candle, your Deity, and the overpowering, all-loving presence of God enveloping you. Feel that your heart is flooded with grace.

Feel that a Divine temple is unfolding within your heart, and in it, seated on a luminous throne, there exists the Divinity—the source of endless love, power, and wisdom. Feel that you are adoring the Divinity and coming closer to His glorious presence.

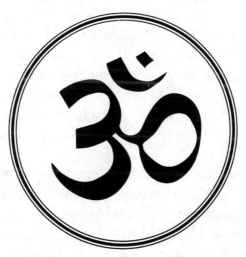

WHAT IS TRUE EDUCATION?

Education is meant to bring out your hidden talents, and to enable you to discover your essential nature and fulfill the purpose of your existence. In so doing you serve humanity in the best way possible. For the vast majority of people, however, the concept of education is extremely limited. People who have big titles or degrees from universities are recognized as educated people and, relatively speaking, that definition is perfectly correct. However, from the point of view of the ideological and philosophical understanding of education, that definition remains shallow. To simply have big degrees, and a lot of recognition and titles does not imply that the person is educated in the true sense.

To be educated, in the more profound sense, implies to be able to develop your human potential and higher human values, to be able to handle your mental stress, to be able to live with people with adaptability, to develop the Divine qualities of the soul: humility, goodness of the heart, compassion, selflessness. If these are lacking, one is not educated.

Let me relate to you a well-known parable: Once a group of scholars entered a boat; one was a mathematician, another was a literary giant, another was a scientist. In the course of conversation, each asked questions of the boatman. The mathematician asked him, "Have you ever read a treatise on mathematics, or have you had any experience with mathematics?" And the boatman said, "No. Just counting some mangoes and vegetables, but nothing beyond that." The mathematician replied, "Then you have lost half of your life since you have never had the joy and the thrill one experiences by possessing mathematical talent." The boatman felt miserable, and said, "What can I do? I was born in a poor family; I could never be educated."

Similarly, the scientist spoke about the wonderful strides taken in physics, in chemistry, in astronomy and so many other branches of science. "Do you have any idea," he asked the boatman, "about the vastness of knowledge in science?" And the boatman said, "No. I am just a poor man." "Then you have lost half of your life by missing so much joy."

And the literary man said, "Have you read Shakespeare or any other great poet? Have you experienced the joy of reading novels?" The boatman replied, "No, I have read nothing. I am illiterate." Now they all pitied him, and he himself felt very miserable.

But as the boat proceeded on its course through the

river, it was caught by a whirlpool that tossed it from side to side. At this point the boatman said, "Do any of you know how to swim? Now we are in a difficult predicament and we may have to jump." And they all replied, "No, we do not know how to swim!" The boatman said, "Well, if that is the case, now all of your lives are gone!"

The moral of this story is that you may have great talents, you may be a computer expert, you may be a great mathematician, you may know how to erect a bridge or build a condominium, but when certain problems develop at home, can you handle them? When you suddenly hear something shocking—the doctor informs you that you have a terminal disease—what happens to your mental balance?

When some challenging situation actually develops in life, all your accomplishments do not come to your aid; then you feel as if you are drowning. On the other hand, there are people who are not so educated from the academic point of view, but they can handle stressing situations, they keep calm in adversity, they have a mature judgement in difficult situations, they can advise others, they radiate a sense of comfort and inspiration for others. Are not these people more educated than so many students that are being manufactured by so many universities year after year?

The educational system, as it was in Vedic times, was geared to enable a student to serve himself and society. Therefore, it was founded on discipline. Anyone who entered the school had to follow the path of *brahmacharya*, which meant a complete discipline of the body, mind, and senses.

In those times, every form of learning was called a *veda*. If you were interested in martial arts you studied *Dhanur Veda*, and you learned archery under a guru who taught you *mantras* (secret formulas) related to archery. First, he disciplined you well and then, when he found you qualified, he taught you archery. If you were interested in medicine, you had to follow the disciplines of *Ayur Veda*. Every branch of knowledge was considered a *veda*, which implied that whatever you were learning you learned with humility and with a spirit of serving God in humanity, always keeping in view the goal of life—Self-realization.

Education and the Four Purposes of Life

In order to understand education in its integral way, you should understand the four purposes of life: *dharma*, *artha*, *kama,* and *Moksha*. *Dharma*, or the cultivation of ethical values, is the basic purpose of life and the foundation of education. All that you achieve and learn should be based on *dharma,* or righteousness. You must possess a clear and sublime conscience. If *dharma* is not there, all your learning is in vain.

If *dharma* is not there, all learning and accomplishment bring about a demoniac development. A person who is undisciplined and unethical may suddenly

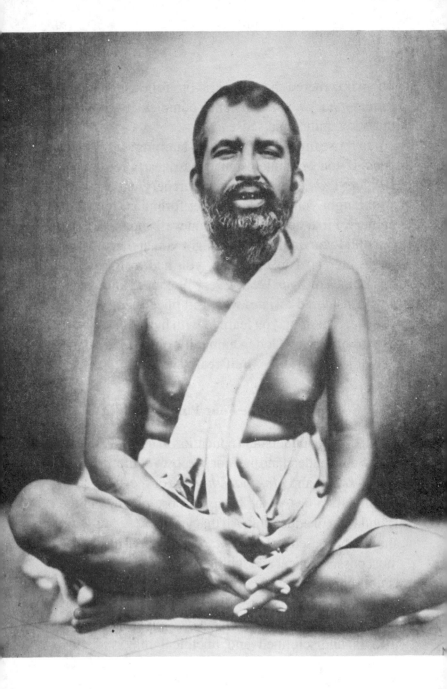

Sri Ramakrishna Paramhamsa

tumble upon an important discovery, and be considered a great man in the eyes of others. However, from a philosophical and spiritual point of view, if his discovery is intended to become a source of misery for others, then that is a demoniac achievement.

Therefore, education must have its roots in *dharma*. The guiding line in an ideal educational system must be to promote harmony and goodness in people. One should never step beyond the principles of nonviolence, truth, and purity. Greed, violence, and passion must not be given license, but are to be controlled.

If a student starts his studies as a doctor, for example, with his mind set upon the idea that "one day I am going to be a millionaire and drive a Rolls Royce," then he is off to a poor start in the light of *dharma*. Although he may set up a wonderful dispensary or hospital, if money is his main inspiration, then his medical attainment is not the product of true education. Although that is the type of education that the majority of people are seeking now, it is not real education.

People crave for pleasure, and pleasure seems to be the goal of the present educational process. Students dream of having lots of money and power—the wealth to go anywhere they want and the resources to own anything they want. However, an education that caters mostly to these values is not education, and an intellect that schemes for these things is called *bhoga buddhi*, an intellect that wants only enjoyment.

There is an ancient saying from the *Mahabharata*: "*Sukharthinah kuto vidya*"—"There is no knowledge for one who loves comfort." If you are a lover of pleasure and comfort, there is no knowledge for you. You are not qualified for education. "*Kuto vidyarthinah sukam*"—"If you are a student, how can there be comfort?" There is no comfort for you if you truly seek knowledge. To shun comfort and luxury is not a miserable development, but rather a joyous development.

Imagine a student who is just twenty-five years old and wants his head propped up by a soft pillow on an easy chair; he doesn't want to do anything but move little buttons on a computer and expects his parents to do all the heavy jobs at home. Outsiders observing the student may think he has become well-educated, but what type of person will he become later? Life presents so many threatening and challenging situations; if one has not been disciplined, if one is not accustomed to hard work, he is ill-prepared to face these challenges.

While teaching children one must not be overprotective and thus spoil the child. If a child is not accustomed to having his ego shaken a little, if he has not developed any patience and endurance in bearing insult and injury, he has not been cultivating *dharma* as the foundation of his education.

The second purpose of life is *artha*, or economic position. Money is a means to a higher end. Just having money does not mean anything at all. Observe how so many people gain millions of dollars overnight in the lottery, yet that doesn't make any difference in the deeper quality of their lives. All the defects in their personalities can even become more exaggerated! This effect is similar to what happens when you look into a magnifying mirror: when there was no magnification, your face looked gentle and fine; but look into a strong magnifying glass and you become a giant and every hair looks like a big pole! That is what suddenly becoming rich can do—it does not in any way make you a better person.

On the other hand, if you are earning money with a basic grounding in *dharma*, then the money that comes to you becomes a means to your self-improvement, a means to helping society by performing good deeds. Used in this manner, it will not stir your vanity.

The next and third purpose of life is *kama*, or developing social relationships. That is also a part of education. If you cannot adapt and adjust to your friends and live in harmony with family members, then life becomes empty.

No matter where you are or in what situation you are placed, you always find the challenge of different relationships. If you cannot handle people with different moods and egocentricities, then life becomes empty.

A person cannot live alone. Even if you were in the Himalayas, you would find that you were making friends with monkeys, birds or squirrels. You would find some relationship to overcome loneliness.

Kama is the vital value of life which allows you to live in harmony with others so that you are then free to plan how to help all humanity. To be able to expand and outgrow one's ego is the most profound aspect of education. A truly educated person is inspired by compassion to help others, and he places every talent he has in the service of others. In that way his talents increase more and more. Selflessness is the secret of discovering more and more talent and abundance within.

Moksha, or Liberation, is the ultimate purpose in life. The entire educational process should lead you to Liberation. In this stage the knowledge that you gain is known as *para vidya*. The *Upanishads* say there are two types of *vidya*, or knowledge: *apara* and *para*.

Apara is the lower knowledge or relative knowledge, the knowledge that helps you in your daily life. Within that category of knowledge comes all the sciences and the arts, all the subjects that are taught in universities. *Para vidya*, however, is the knowledge that is mystical. When you practise concentration and meditation and are guided by a *guru*, then you discover a knowledge which brings about a complete fulfillment of the urge to know. *Para vidya* is that knowledge by which all is known.

Para vidya is the attainment in which all educational systems must culminate. That is the goal. Keeping this in view, an ideal student should develop self-discipline; he should strive to develop virtuous qualities like humility, patience, sincerity, and simplicity; he should practise self-introspection and austerity; he should be self-dependent; he should flow out of himself in service to humanity and thereby commune with God. These are the great highlights of true education. If you have these, you are really educated. Anything other than this is a deviation—lack of education. May God bless you with the purity of intellect that leads you to health, long life, peace, prosperity, success, and Liberation!

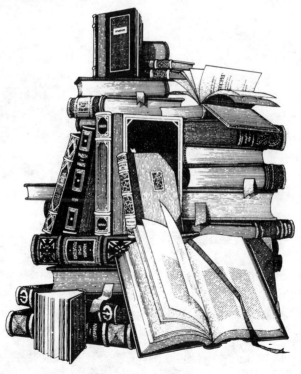

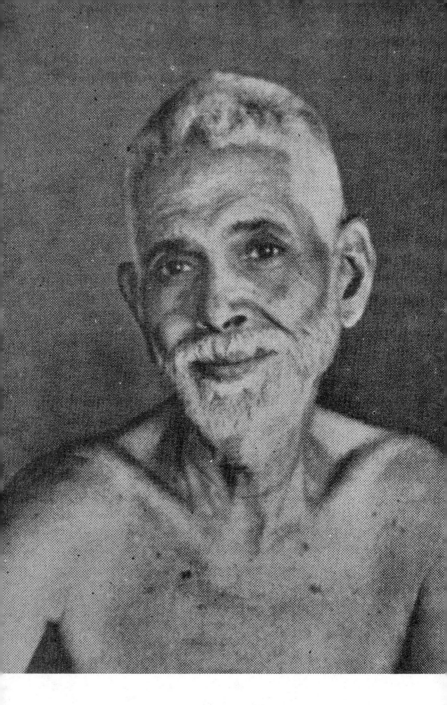

Sri Ramana Maharshi

3

UNFOLDING POSITIVE QUALITIES

If
you pursue
the path of virtue,
victory will be yours!

A DIVINE TREASURE HUNT

You must be as enthusiastic about cultivating positive qualities as you would be about discovering a buried treasure of jewels and gold. Day by day, little by little, try to develop as many virtues as you can. Even if you fail a thousand times, still you should continue with sincere effort.

Never doubt for a moment the power of positive thinking. The daily repetition of strong positive affirmations will help you overcome the negative within your personality and enhance any virtue you sincerely wish to develop.

Keep a list of virtues prominently posted in your room. Each time you look at them, your heart will be filled with good thoughts. Be sure to include the following virtues on your list:

Nonviolence   Fearlessness
Humility   Straightforwardness

Truthfulness	Forgiveness
Endurance	Generosity
Compassion	Friendliness
Cheerfulness	Presence of Mind
Simplicity	Purity

The first step in developing your virtuous qualities is to look at yourself with an open mind. Do you see any of the following negative qualities in your personality: anger, hatred, pride, hypocrisy, falsehood, fear, greed, violence, cruelty, harsh speech, gossiping nature, jealousy, lust or passion?

If so, the next step is to determine what virtue is opposite to that negative quality and try to cultivate it. For example, suppose you realize that you are unable to control your speech, and you find yourself saying many things which you shouldn't say. Make an internal resolve: "I will control my irritability and master my speech." Work towards this goal for one week, reminding yourself again and again of the benefits of possessing that virtue and trying your best to express it in your daily life.

The next week focus your attention on some other negative quality and work on it in a similar manner. By doing this you will gradually eliminate the negative within you and cultivate the positive. As you take up one virtue after another in this way, you will begin to truly enjoy the challenge of this "treasure hunt" for Divine qualities!

A Transforming Pranayama

In Section Six of this book, you are introduced to an important yogic breathing exercise called *Sukha Purvaka Pranayama*, or alternate nostril breathing. *Sukha Purvaka Pranayama* is very effective in arousing the mystic powers of the spirit. If you maintain a positive mental attitude while practising the exercise, it can help you to unfold the Divine qualities latent in your personality.

Study the method of performing this exercise as explained on page 221. When you have memorized the directions for inhaling, retaining, and exhaling, and feel comfortable with the exercise, close your eyes and practise this powerful *pranayama* with the following mental attitude:

As you inhale, feel that the qualities associated with a particular virtue are being showered upon you like spring rains bathing the dry earth; as you retain, feel that your deep unconscious is being flooded with the joyous impressions of that quality; as you exhale, feel that you are ridding yourself of any unconscious negative impressions that oppose the virtue.

Practise this *pranayama* several times during the day. Each time you do so, positive impressions for change will flourish within your heart.

Just as darkness cannot exist when there is light, so too, vice cannot exist when virtue is developed. By regular effort and strong resolve, you will succeed in eradicating all that is negative within you, and the jewels of Divine virtues will shine forth and illumine your path.

WHO IS A HERO
IN THE BATTLE OF LIFE?

Since life is a constant battle—the battle between the forces of light and the forces of darkness—heroism is needed at every moment in your life. In order to be a spiritual hero, you must be endowed with willpower and insight, you must learn the art of controlling the senses, and you must live a life that is illumined by reason.

To be a spiritual hero you must wear the armor of Divine impressions created by the repetition of *mantra* (Divine name) and prayer. As you move in the battle-field of the world, there are arrows of negativity, sorrow and grief that fly at you from every direction. If you are not shielding yourself with the armor of inner power generated by repetition of *mantra* and prayer, you are vulnerable to attack.

To be a hero you must hold the shield of Divine Grace and march on the path of righteous conduct. Your sword is your sharp, penetrating intellect that slays the enemy forces of darkness. Each time egoism, greed, and hatred raise their heads, you must slay them with the subtle sword of reason.

Pure intellect is like a supersonic jet that carries you high above the realm of ego. When you practise meditation and enquiry into "Who am I?" you are dropping a bomb on the city of the enemy where ignorance dwells.

Your clear mind is your gun, and powerful thoughts are the bullets. When your mind is filled with Divine thoughts, you can easily destroy all the enemies of the soul!

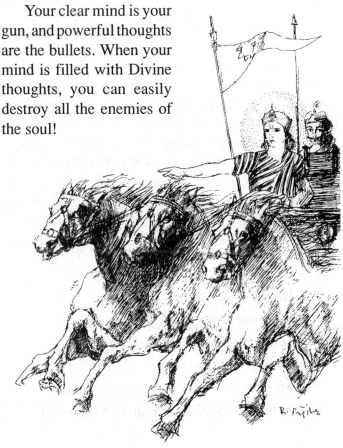

TEN SECRETS FOR LIVING A VIRTUOUS LIFE

Dharma, ordinarily translated as virtue or righteousness or ethical conduct, has many implications and is a most significant term in Hindu culture and philosophy. The scriptures say, *"Yato Dharmas Tato Jaya"*—"Wherever there is *dharma* there is victory."

Great Sage Manu gave ten characteristics of *dharma* in *Manu Smriti*, a Hindu scripture. These ten are referred to as *Dharma Lakshanas*. In fact, they are the basis for righteousness in every religion of the world. One should meditate upon these characteristics and try to develop them:

- **Dhriti** – Firmness
- **Kshama** – Forgiveness, forbearance
- **Dama** – Control of the senses
- **Asteya** – Nonstealing
- **Shaucha** – Purity of body and mind
- **Atma Vinigraha** – Control of the mind

- **Dhee** – Purity of intellect
- **Vidya** – Knowledge
- **Satya** – Truthfulness
- **Akrodha** – Absence of anger

1. DHRITI—FIRMNESS

Dhriti means firmness or persistence. If you make a resolve to accomplish something, then come what may, you should be able to pursue that project to its completion. Even if someone criticizes you or tries to discourage you, do not be affected; rather, move on towards your goal in an undaunted manner.

Dhriti is especially important when you are doing something good, for that is when you should never allow yourself to become discouraged. In pursuing what is good you must be firm and strong.

However, you should not be firm about pursuing negative things. If your friends become lazy or start smoking or begin to use drugs, then do not pursue that with them. Firmness is for positive things.

The Transformation of Kalidas

I will give you a humorous story that shows the power of *dhriti*:

Kalidas is known as one of the greatest scholars of Sanskrit literature, but in his early days he was more dull-witted than you can imagine! When he was a young man, there was a highly intelligent princess in his country who had acquired much literary and scriptural knowledge, and had become a great Sanskrit scholar. When she reached the age for marriage, her father announced that only someone whose knowledge was equal to or greater than hers could become her husband.

Many young scholars came to try to win her hand, but she defeated them all in philosophical discussions. Some suitors who felt particularly humiliated and upset by this defeat decided to teach her a lesson. So, they put their heads together and plotted to find an extremely stupid person and trick the princess into marrying him.

During their search, they found a good-looking young man who was sitting on a branch of a tree, busily cutting the same branch upon which he was seated! They realized that here was the stupidest man they could hope to find. So they beckoned him to come down and asked him if he would like to marry the princess. He loved the idea, but asked how it could possibly happen. They told him that all that he would have to do was to keep quiet and not

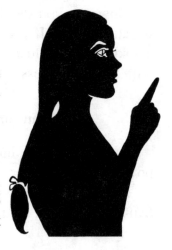

speak a word. However, he could make all the gestures he wanted with his hands.

So, these people brought the dull-wit into the palace and presented him in the royal court as the greatest philosopher and sage of the time. They said that he was so advanced that he didn't even have to use words. In silence, just by gestures, he could convey the highest philosophy. They challenged the princess to debate with him in the same language of silent gestures, or else accept defeat.

The princess accepted the challenge, and they both sat down, ready to begin the unusual debate. The princess raised one finger, implying, "Can you refute that there is only one God, one Absolute?"

The dull-wit, seeing that raised finger, thought that the princess was going to poke his eye. So he thought, "Let me poke both of hers." And he raised two fingers.

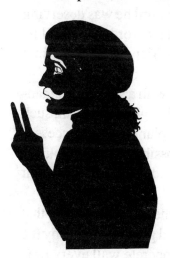

The scheming scholars interpreted this for the princess, saying, "O princess, our scholar friend is more advanced than you are. Although *Brahman* is One, one alone cannot create and sustain this world. *Brahman* must have *maya* (cosmic illusion) to do so." Hearing this, the princess accepted defeat on this point and went on to another.

She then raised her hand showing five fingers, implying that the world is made up of five elements, or five *tattwas*. Seeing her hand raised, this dull-wit thought that she was going to slap him. He said to himself, "If she tries to slap me, I am going to punch her!" So he made a fist.

The philosophers interpreted this, saying, "The princess asserts that five elements make the world. But if the five elements are apart like her fingers, how can those elements go to form the world? This sage is advanced. With his fist he shows that the five elements must come together." The princess again had to accept defeat.

In this way, those scholars succeeded in getting the young man married to the princess. It was not difficult, however, for the princess to find out that he was indeed a dull-wit. The moment she realized this she told him to get out and not to come back until he was deserving of being married to her—in other words, not until he became the scholar that all his friends had made him out to be.

So, that young man left her with a sense of tremendous sorrow. Deeply hurt, he thought, "I who am such a dull-wit, how can I be the scholar that the princess is expecting me to be? It is impossible." Thus thinking, he sat down by a well with the idea of jumping into it to commit suicide.

But as he sat looking into the well, he noticed that the walls had deeply entrenched grooves, made by the rope as it rubbed against the concrete wall every time people drew water. So, he thought to himself, "If by persistent rubbing even concrete gives way and changes, what will happen to my mind if I persist? I do want to be a scholar, well-cultured and intelligent. So why can't I, too, change?" With that resolve he became a devotee of Goddess Kali, and with sustained perseverance began studying under a great scholar. Eventually he became Kalidas—one of the greatest poets, writers, dramatists, and literary scholars of the Sanskrit language.

That firmness of resolve is what we refer to as *dhriti*. If you set your mind to something and refuse to be discouraged, you are bound to succeed. The eternal Self or Spirit within you is inexhaustible in Its energy and resources. Nothing is impossible for you.

Books of ordinary psychology may tell you that your mind can advance only to a certain extent. But that is not so. There is no limit to your capacity. If you know the subtle mystic art, you can bring out amazing talents and powers from within yourself.

With *dhriti,* you develop a strong-metalled personality and strive to accomplish your goals, regardless of the obstacles along the way, and no matter what the odds against your success. If things do not turn out the way you expect, you do not relent, but patiently continue to put forth your best effort. With persistence, eventually you will succeed.

There is another special type of firmness or *dhriti* that helps you translate theoretical knowledge into practical knowledge. If you lack this type of *dhriti*, you hear wonderful things through one ear but they pass right out through the other!

Parable of the Three Skulls

Once a man brought three skulls before a great king and posed a riddle: Which of the three was the wisest when alive? All the great scholars and philosophers in the court looked at the skulls and said that they could not say which one was the wisest just by seeing the skull.

However, one philosopher took the skulls and tried a demonstration with three straws. He poked the first straw into the ear of the first skull and let it pass out through the other ear. At this, the philosopher said, "This one was the dullest. Whatever he listened to in one ear passed right out the other."

Then he poked the second straw into the ear of the second skull and he let it pass out through the mouth. He said, "This one was of medium class wisdom. He heard so many things, but he just went on talking about what he had learned without assimilating any of it."

Then he poked the third straw into the third skull and let it pass through the ear down towards the stomach. "This man was the wisest," said the philosopher. "He digested and assimilated all that he learned."

The story shows that if you have developed *dhriti,* you possess the type of mind that listens, retains, and assimilates. *Dhriti* should be of a *satwic* (pure) nature.

You should be able to retain that which is sublime, not that which is *rajasic* (impure) or *tamasic* (dull). If you have *dhriti*, then whatever you learn will become effective in your life. If you lack *dhriti*, you simply learn things theoretically, but that theoretical knowledge is never put into practice.

2. KSHAMA—FORGIVENESS

Kshama means forgiveness or forbearance. Even when you are placed in a provocative situation, continue to maintain a mind that is serene, without developing ill will towards those who provoke you.

For example, when a doctor approaches a patient, that patient, due to mental imbalance, may say many harsh things to the doctor. The doctor doesn't care. The doctor knows that because his patient is ill, he will shout, cry, and be impatient. These are the expressions of his disease. So therefore, no matter how badly the patient may behave, the doctor continues to try to help him. That same mature attitude must characterize all your dealings with other people. No matter what happens, there must be constant forbearance.

The Drowning Scorpion

Once a saintly person entered into a river and found a scorpion drowning. As he tried to rescue the scorpion, the animal stung him. His hand shook from the pain, and the scorpion fell. Again he tried to pick it up, and again the scorpion stung him.

Someone by the bank of the river laughed at the saint, saying, "Why are you doing this? Throw that scorpion down. Crush it." The saint replied, "The scorpion is maintaining his *dharma* (duty), which is to go on stinging me. Why should I not maintain my *dharma*, which is to go on trying to protect him?"

Similarly, in this world you face different types of personalities, some of which sting like scorpions. No matter how you try to help them, you get stung! Still, you must maintain your *dharma* (duty). Don't use your energy to judge the actions of others, nor to decide what they should or should not do. Rather, look within yourself, decide how you should act, and then do so. *"Yato dharmas tato jayah"* —"Where there is *dharma,* or righteousness, there is victory." If you have forbearance, you will find that people around you will change for the better, and that the change will be of a lasting nature.

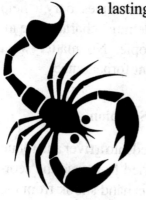

If you want to be great, you must understand that there are two types of strength: strength of muscles and strength of ethics. Strength of ethics implies doing what is good, even when you are provoked, all the while knowing that God is behind that strength.

The Monkeys and the Bull

Buddhist literature tells how Lord Buddha attained perfection passing through many embodiments. In each embodiment he learned a lesson. In one of his incarnations, Buddha was a mighty bull in a forest—and although a bull, his spirit was highly elevated.

One day, a band of wild monkeys began to tease him. Some jumped around on his back; some started scratching his ears; some bit his horns; some played with his tail, etc.

At first the bull thought, "Let me shake those pesty creatures off and crush them." But then he reflected more deeply upon the matter and thought, "After all, these monkeys are having fun, and I am not going to die from all this. They are simply annoying me. If I retaliate they will be seriously injured. Furthermore, isn't it better to control anger than to take revenge?" By reflecting in this manner, the bull was able to remain quietly passive and overpower his anger.

At that moment, some celestial beings passing by observed the conduct of the bull and were amazed! They said to the bull, "Why don't you kill those monkeys?" And the bull said, "It would be easy for me to kill them, but I realize that there is greater virtue in controlling anger. It is a better form of heroism to kill anger than to revenge upon others. Those monkeys have given me the opportunity of discovering my strength over my own lower self. Because of this, I am indebted to the monkeys."

As the story implies, physical strength is little compared to moral strength, to the strength of virtue. And that moral strength develops when you control expressions of anger, hate, and retaliation.

If someone insults you, instead of trying to hurt the person or to revenge upon him, try to maintain goodwill. If you can talk with the person and make him understand, that would be ideal. But if you cannot reason with the person, then simply pray in silence for his well-being. No matter what happens, learn the art of endurance, and internally do not hold any ill will.

It is easy for anybody in the world to follow the philosophy of "tit-for-tat" or "an eye for an eye and a tooth for a tooth"—to revenge upon anyone who harms you. But it is a greater virtue not to seek revenge, but to endure and forgive through the development of inner strength.

If you restrain anger, hate, and jealousy and instead promote compassion, understanding, and love, you become a highly advanced person. The capacity to forgive is a mark of internal greatness. But, if you react in the same way as the average person, you remain at a very low level— for there is no end to taking revenge. The disharmony continues without end.

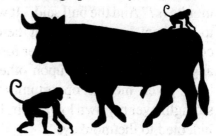

3. DAMA—CONTROL
OF THE SENSES

Dama means control or mastery of the senses, which implies utilizing the senses under the direction of reason. Mastery of the senses does not mean that the senses remain constantly withdrawn. In order to be useful in this practical world, the senses have to operate in a healthy and sensitive way. However, you must be vigilant as to when you should withdraw them and when you should not. The senses must always be under the control of your reason.

There is a popular expression: "See no evil, hear no evil, think no evil." Even when you are seeing evil, you have the possibility of not letting the evil enter your mind. When you hear negative things, you have the possibility of rejecting the impressions that are carried through those words.

Dama also implies disciplining the senses so they can be utilized in the right direction at the right time. When it is time to study, you must do so, without being distracted by what the senses bring before you. When it is time to play, you should play fully. You should not just pursue things haphazardly according to your whims.

A person who is fabulously rich may have millions of dollars in his hands, but he may be no more than a slave to his senses. Although he has a lot of money, his desires may be endless. He may run from one place to another, a slave to a thousand fancies. He may decide to have breakfast in Paris, lunch in New York, and dinner in Australia. His life becomes as scattered as his senses.

If you are undisciplined, your senses become your worst enemies. When you discipline yourself, you find you can do so many things in an excellent manner. Discipline, order, and harmony—these are the secrets of real success in your life. All the pleasure that the senses can give are little compared to the joy that arises when your mind advances and you have attained mastery over the senses. The Bliss of the Self is like the ocean. All the pleasures of the senses are just a drop in that ocean.

The Search for a Contented Goat

Once a king issued a declaration that if any farmer brought to him a truly contented goat, he would give that farmer a wonderful reward. Throughout the kingdom, farmers prepared for that competition by feeding their goats special food for months.

On the appointed day, the goats were brought to the stage one by one and their contentedness was tested as fresh green grass was held before their noses. Although each goat was already strong and well-fed, tempted by the luscious grass each one lost control and started eating as if he had not eaten before—and one by one they failed the test!

Then one farmer came forward with a goat that was not as fat and stout looking as the others. Looking at that goat, the other farmers never thought that he was much of a competitor. But then something quite unexpected happened. The goat looked eagerly at the grass, but before he could move toward it, he looked at his master as he had been well trained to do. The master raised a little cane rod. Seeing this, the goat turned away from the grass and wouldn't eat. By so doing, he passed the examination and got the reward.

Similarly, your senses are like goats. No matter how much you give them, they are never pleased. You may eat all the ice cream in the world, but you will still want more. You may have hours of fun but still you will want more fun. The senses are never satisfied.

You must, then, use the rod of your discrimination, of your intellect. Tell your senses, you can have half an hour more of fun but that's all! You can have one more bowl of ice cream, but that's all! As you begin to discipline yourself, you build the foundation for a wonderful personality.

Later in life, when you have learned the value of discipline, you are grateful that your parents helped you to discipline yourself when you were young. But when you grow up undisciplined, you feel that your parents didn't do their duty to help you as much as they should have.

The Resentful Thief

A story is told about a child who used to steal pencils from his classmates and bring them to his mother. The mother always seemed happy to get the pencils, which encouraged the child to steal more and more. As the child grew up he continued to steal, and eventually the police arrested him for more serious theft and sentenced him to prison.

Before the thief was to be imprisoned, he asked permission to see his mother. When she was brought before him, he went close to her ear as if he wanted to whisper something to her privately. Instead of speaking, however, he bit her ear! In surprise she cried out, "Why are you doing this to me? Haven't I always been a loving mother to you ?" The son replied, "That's just the problem, mother. Why didn't you slap me the very first time I stole the pencils? Why didn't you discipline me rather than encourage me? Why didn't you help me understand the importance of restraining myself?"

Regulate Your Life

The secret of controlling the senses lies in your mind. When you work towards a goal, your mind must be filled with determination: "This is what I want to do, and I will do it."

Suppose, for example, that you are preparing for an exam, and there is only one week left. Plan your time so that a certain amount of work will be accomplished every day, and follow the plan with patience. Do not become hysterical, thinking, "Oh, what can I do? I haven't studied enough. The exam is only a few days away!" When you become hysterical, what you have learned flies right out of your mind.

Rather, plan things well and have patience. If you have disciplined senses, you will go on following your plan and will feel confident at the time of your exam.

Controlling the senses means regulating your life: knowing when to sleep and when to get up; knowing how to schedule your activities so that day by day you accomplish something important. When the senses are not controlled, your mind constantly becomes distracted from its goals and it is difficult for you to accomplish anything significant in your life.

In the *Gita*, Lord Krishna says that you should be harmonized in eating, in fasting, in playing, and in sleeping. Include everything that is necessary in your life, but in a balanced way. Do not go overboard. Be moderate in everything you do and always have a goal before you.

The energy of your mind and senses is like sunlight. Sunlight is diffused everywhere, but if you focus that sunlight through a lens it can start a fire and bring forth a flame. Similarly, energy is scattered in your mind; but when you learn how to focus your mental energy by disciplining your senses, you develop a power by which you can achieve anything.

4. ASTEYA—NONSTEALING

Every ethical person knows that stealing is immoral and it should not be done. However, there are subtler forms of stealing that many people never reflect upon. If you hoard more than you need, if you come in the way of somebody's progress or take away other people's opportunities, or if you acquire something by adopting immoral or illegal methods, that is also stealing.

The urge to steal results from a blend of greed and lack of control over senses. Therefore, to be established in *asteya,* or nonstealing, one must learn to discipline the senses and root out the subtlest forms of greed.

The secret of abundance is not to be greedy. If you do not have a greedy mind, you will have an abundance of things. If you become established in *asteya* to a great degree, Raja Yoga says, all the wealth of the world will be drawn to you.

5. SHAUCHA—
PURITY OF BODY AND MIND

Purity is of two types: physical and mental. Physical purity refers to matters of personal hygiene and health. You must keep yourself clean by taking baths and washing your clothes. Physical purity also involves observing laws of health. You may wear the cleanest clothes but, internally, if you are filling your body with toxins from junk food or other impure foods, then you are not promoting true physical health or purity.

Eating *satwic* or pure food is very important for keeping you free from illness and for giving you energy and happiness. If you want to promote physical purity, you must evolve a lifestyle that allows your body to remain healthy through good diet, plenty of exercise, and sufficient rest.

Mental purity implies being free of negative thoughts of lust, greed, anger, hate, pride, jealousy, etc. These negative qualities make your mind impure. Mental purity is even more important than physical purity.

Instead of negative thoughts try to cultivate positive thoughts. Just as a house needs to be cleaned every day, in the same way, the mind needs to be cleaned.

And how do you clean the mind? You do that by *satsanga,* or good association. When you come to listen to spiritual teachings, when you associate with people who are calm and harmonious, and when you read the elevating words of sages and saints, your mind becomes pure.

Saint Kabira and the Pigs

Once some Islamic priests challenged Kabira—a great saint and poet of sixteenth century India—to a debate on spiritual matters. Kabira accepted and told the students to come to his home on a certain day.

On that day, prior to the group's arrival, Kabira tied up some pigs right in front of his door. He had done this deliberately, knowing how Islamic priests hate pigs. When they came and saw those pigs in their path, they became terribly upset. Speaking abusively, they shouted, "O shame, shame that Kabira is so full of mud and dirt that he keeps pigs in front of his door."

From inside the house, Kabira, who was expecting this reaction from the priests, called out: "I have tied my pigs outside, but you have tied your pigs inside— within your mind."

As the story implies, anger, greed,

and jealousy are like pigs tied up within the mind. You may have a wonderful house and garden, with everything kept perfectly clean and neat. Yet, if your mind harbors selfishness and hypocrisy, it is as if pigs were everywhere, causing dirty and unhealthy conditions.

Thus, purity must be practised on both levels—physical and mental. If you have mental purity, you will enjoy serenity, harmony, and cheerfulness. There is a subtle link between your mind and your body. The moment a negative thought enters your mind, it sets up a discordant vibration in the *pranas,* or vital forces, in your body. The moment the vital forces are disharmonized, there is an imbalance in the assimilation of what you have eaten. Nutrition becomes disturbed and one portion of your body receives more nourishment and another less. So even though your overall health may be good, your liver may become sick, or your heart may become weakened and ultimately your entire body will suffer from the effects of mental stress and tension.

Your mind, in addition to directly influencing the well-being of your body, creates *karmas*. Through those *karmas* you are drawing circumstances and situations to yourself—good or bad. Therefore, purifying the mind, or keeping it free of anger, hate, greed, and other disturbing sentiments is of vital importance in your life.

6. ATMA VINIGRAHA—
CONTROL OF THE MIND

Mind is more miraculous than Aladdin's lamp. Through your mind, you can do amazing things. However, mind needs to be constantly watched, observed and disciplined to tap its immense powers.

In most people, mental energy is constantly wasted through distraction. If you watch your mind, you will probably discover that you can't keep your mind truly focused on anything for more than two or three minutes.

If you learn the art of concentration, you will begin to realize the hidden powers of your mind. Through the benefits of concentration, you will be able to handle stressing situations successfully, you will develop memory power, you will be able to work more systematically, you will save a lot of time, you will have greater in-depth comprehension in your studies and knowledge of many things will reveal itself to you automatically.

In the mind that is distracted, two forces constantly are fighting with each other. One wants to go this way and the other wants to go that way. Discordant and contrary thoughts keep you from experiencing your innate mental strength. A story is told that illustrates that point:

The Magic Mat

Once there was a person who practised intense austerity and meditation. As a result of this, one day a deity appeared before him and gave him a magic mat. The magic mat had special powers: whatever was thought about by anyone sitting on the mat would come true.

So the man took the magic mat, sat upon it, and thought about having wonderful food. Immediately, golden platters of food appeared before him and he felt so joyous.

Then he thought to himself, "All right, why shouldn't I wish for more than this? Wouldn't it be nice if I had a wonderful palace?" Then, quick as a wink, the palace appeared before him.

Then he thought about having servants and many other people around him to bring good fellowship to the palace—and his wish was immediately fulfilled.

No sooner had he begun enjoying all that the mat had provided, than a strange thought suddenly arose in his mind: "What would happen to his palace if there were an earthquake?" And immediately there was an earthquake and the whole palace collapsed upon him.

Your mind is like that magic mat. Through your good thoughts you accomplish a great deal, but then, from your unconscious, come thoughts of fear and insecurity, and what you have accomplished is destroyed. In this way, the strength of your mind is never fully realized and experienced.

However there are concentration techniques to help you solve this problem and learn to focus and channel your mental energy. Those techniques involve prayer, *japa* (repetition of Divine name), meditation, and reflection. These practices give you increased mental strength day by day.

7. DHEE—PURITY OF INTELLECT

Intellect is the greatest power within you, the driving force in the chariot of human personality. But intellect becomes clouded by egoism, by desire, by anger. Thus, intellect must be kept pure.

In the world of practical realities, it is through intellect that you understand things clearly and profoundly. When you do not understand things well, problems are created. When you have correct understanding, problems become little and you can solve them easily.

The Rabbit That Used His Intellect

Once in a forest there was a greedy lion who hunted and killed the other animals indiscriminately, often killing more than he was able to eat. The animals were filled with terror, and feared that they would all be eliminated from their forest home unless something was done about the situation.

So the animals held a meeting and came up with a proposal that they hoped the lion would accept. Appearing humbly before the lion, a spokesman for the animals said, "O lion king, we want to save you all the work of hunting for your food. So each day we will bring right to your doorstep one animal from among us for your meal. In return, you must promise not to kill any other animals that day."

"All right," said the lion. "I will agree as long as my food arrives at my door every day on time."

So the new plan went into effect. Each day, one animal was chosen to be the lion's food, and the lion was content and harmony was again established in the forest.

Soon the turn came for the rabbit to be sacrificed as food for the lion. But that rabbit loved his life intensely and he just could not accept the idea of giving it up so easily. So he thought and thought and thought and, using his keen intelligence, came up with a clever plan.

While the rabbit was thinking, the lion was getting hungrier and hungrier, waiting angrily by his door for his next meal to arrive. Finally the rabbit appeared, walking quickly toward him.

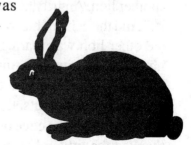

"Where have you been, you stupid rabbit? Why do you come so late?" The rabbit said, "I had a frightening adventure on the way. As I was walking here, I met another lion who said that he was king of the forest, and he was going to eat me up. But I pleaded saying, 'Do not eat me up yet. Let me go and report this to my king and then I'll come back to you.' So that lion agreed and allowed me to come to you."

"What!" the lion roared. "Who is this impostor who says he is king? Let me meet him and show him who is king!" The rabbit replied, "I will show you where this impostor is if you want to see him. Follow me."

And so the clever little rabbit led the lion through the forest until they came to a clearing where there was an old well. Then the rabbit said, "Look inside and you will see that lion who was claiming to be king of the forest."

So, without much thought, the lion put his head down into the well, and when he saw his own reflection in the water, he was convinced that he was seeing another lion. Angrily he roared, "There he is! There he is!" And the echo of his own voice made him think that the other lion was roaring at him. Eager to fight that impostor, he jumped into the well—and quickly drowned in the cold water.

Hearing the shouts, the other animals of the forest had gathered at the edge of the well. They rejoiced and thanked the little rabbit who had used his intellect to rescue himself and to bring peace and harmony back to their homes.

Similarly, when you use your intellect, things that are ordinarily impossible become possible. When you grow in wisdom and exercise your intellect in the right direction, you can be of great service to yourself and to humanity.

Purity of intellect should be promoted by all your academic studies; however, it is especially promoted by study of the scriptures. Learn to meditate upon what the scriptures say. Try to figure out, "Who am I?" Try to understand what the sages mean when they say, "You are not the body. You are the soul that is immortal. You do not have to be afraid of anything. The real you is not affected by what happens to the body—even death does not destroy the real you." By training your intellect you will eventually begin to understand these points.

Purity of intellect is more important than intellectualism. You can be a great intellectual, but if you do not have purity of intellect you will not be able to control your mind and enjoy inner peace. There are so many professors with impressive degrees—but they cannot control their tempers, their moods, their uncertainties, their fears.

Intellect must be able to grasp higher truth. Once it does so, your whole personality begins to change. That is why so much importance has been given to the Vedic prayer called *Gayatri Mantra:*

"Om bhur bhuvah swah, tat savitur varenyam, bhargo devasya dhimahi, dhiyo yo naha pra-chodayat."—"We adore God, Who is like the shining sun, Who permeates the three planes (physical, astral, and causal). May He enlighten our intellects."

Prayer for enlightenment of the intellect is the highest prayer. You need not pray for anything else. All is possible once your intellect is enlightened.

8. VIDYA—KNOWLEDGE

Knowledge is of two types: *apara-vidya* and *para-vidya*. All the academic knowledge that allows you to carry on your practical affairs in the world of time and space—the knowledge of geography, history, language, science, mathematics, arts, etc.—is called *apara* or "lower" knowledge.

The academic knowledge that you acquire from schools and colleges is only a means to an end. There is a much greater knowledge to be acquired as you live your life: how to handle frustration, how to handle an unexpected adversity, how to steer your life through the turmoils of the world, how to attain your goals in spite of obstacles. That type of knowledge is spiritual knowledge, which you acquire through *satsanga,* or good association, by listening to advanced people and reflecting upon their teachings.

It is this spiritual knowledge which eventually blossoms into the highest knowledge, which is referred to as *para-vidya*. *Para-vidya* is intuitional knowledge of the Self, the knowledge that grants you Liberation—that knowledge by which all else is known.

Liberation is the goal of life. It is called *Mukti* by the yogis, *Nirvana* by the Buddhists, and the Kingdom of Heaven by the Christians. The knowledge that leads you to that stage—which makes you internally free of all defects of mind and leads you to internal communion with God—is called *para-vidya*.

One must possess both types of knowledge. The lower type of knowledge that you gain is a means to the development of spiritual knowledge. Whatever you have learned in schools and universities and whatever talents you have cultivated must enable you to serve humanity and to advance in a spiritual way towards intuitional knowledge.

9. SATYA—TRUTHFULNESS

Always understand that the truth wins. No one can hide the truth. Even if it is only whispered, that whisper one day will gain tremendous force. Falsehood, even if it is shouted and broadcast through all the TV's all over the world, will dwindle.

The Chinese King's Secret

There was once a Chinese king who had a secret. He had a strange looking horn on his head and he didn't want it to be seen by anyone. So he went to his barber (who in those days also did surgical work) and asked him to remove it. After the operation was successfully completed, the king made the barber pledge that he would never tell anyone about the horn that he had removed.

The barber agreed, but it was against his nature to keep a secret for more than a few days. Unable to bear it any longer, he went out into the forest, dug a hole, put his mouth into the hole and said, "The king had a horn on his head." And then he covered it up and went away.

Soon the grass began to grow over the hole and then the field was full of grass swaying in the wind. And as the wind blew, a sound came from the grass: "The King of China had a horn on his head!" And everyone came to know about the strange secret.

Similarly, you cannot hide anything in this world. Nature has a way of bringing everything out. Many families hide their secrets in a closet—without realizing that sometimes the closet opens up! In this mysterious world, God knows everything. Therefore, you must develop great sincerity within yourself.

Satya is more the practice of internal sincerity than of speaking factually. Be sincere to yourself and automatically your dealings with others will become more sincere.

Truth is to be practised in various levels—in your thinking, in your speech, in your actions. Learning to speak the truth is not as simple as it may seem. For example, suppose somebody has a personality defect and, in the name of truth, you point it out in such a way that people laugh at that person. The result will be animosity and anger. Or suppose there is a flea on your classmate's nose, or there is some mud on his chin. If you say in an abrupt way, "Now, look at your dirty face!" the boy will become embarrassed. It would be better to let him know in a way that does not hurt his feelings.

There is a saying in Sanskrit: *"Satyam vada priyam vada na vada satyam apriyam."*—"Speak the truth, but not to hurt others' feelings. The truth that you speak should be pleasing to others."

You should plan your words carefully so that others are glad to hear the truth and are not hurt by it. If by speaking the truth you are hurting others, then you are not speaking the truth. If your intention is to hurt others, that is violence disguised in the form of truth. Truth is practised for the purpose of realizing God, not for fulfilling the demands of ego.

More important than merely speaking the truth is practising the truth through your actions. Internally look within yourself and see whether you are practising what you believe, what you say.

There must be harmony between your thoughts, words, and actions. Think truly, speak truly, act truly. A person who expresses the truth on all these levels becomes a dynamic personality. He is a blossoming flower in the tree of society. Mahatma Gandhi prac-

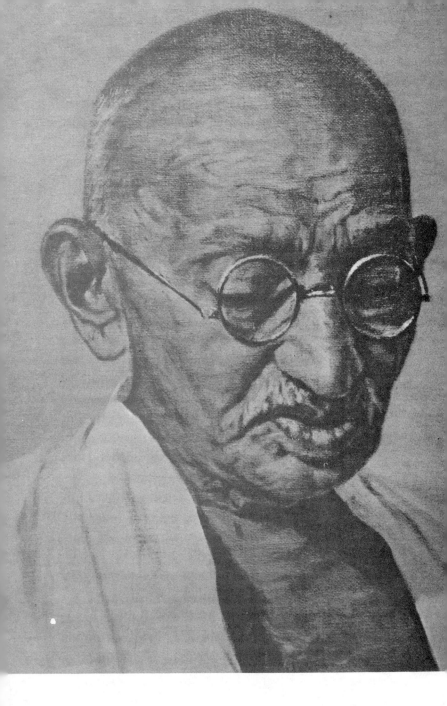

Mahatma Gandhi

tised truth, nonviolence and *brahmacharya* (sex-restraint). These are the greatest qualities.

Do not cheat yourself. If you discover that repetition of *mantra* helps you, then sincerely try to practise it. If you discover that faith in God has great power, then strive to develop more of it. When you simply talk about things that you know to be important without practising them, that is lack of truth.

Sincerity is the secret of all success and prosperity. If you are sincere and people come to know of this, they will be drawn to you like iron filings are drawn to a magnet. Sincere people exert great influence on society. Insincere people may make a great splash for a while, but they cannot succeed in the long run. The world has been fashioned in such a way that truth eventually triumphs: *"Satyameva jayate naanritam"* — "Truth alone triumphs, not falsehood."

10. AKRODA—ABSENCE OF ANGER OR AGITATION

Once there was a judge who had the habit of always becoming angry. One day he realized that his anger had become a great problem and he told his servant, "Whenever I become angry, bring a mirror and put it in front of my face." The servant replied, "Well, if I put the mirror before you, I will become the target of your anger." The judge said, "No, I give you my word."

So each time the judge became angry, his servant brought the mirror before him; each time the judge saw how ugly his face became when it was distorted by anger, he tried a little harder to control it!

Once you develop disgust towards anger you are well on the road to controlling it. Once you begin to realize it should not be there, you begin to learn the art of dominating it.

Not only should you not become angry yourself, but you should not agitate or provoke others to anger. Do not bring out from others their lesser qualities, but exert your influence to bring out the best in others.

When you see older people angry, you become upset. You may think to yourself, "Why is my aunt always angry? Why is my grandfather irritable? Why does my father shout at everybody when nothing has really happened?"

Many people who are slaves to anger allow their intellect to justify it. How often have you heard someone say, "If I do not become angry, how will things get done? How can the children be trained? How can the servants work? How can people be kept in their place if I don't become angry?" The fact is, all those things can happen even if you develop calmness of mind—and in a much better way! Without ever looking down upon those who cannot control themselves, you must understand what leads to that development.

When you are young, it seems more fun not to discipline yourself, to let your emotions roll by uncontrolled. But when you get older, all that is undisciplined in your personality is distilled down by the mind, and it becomes so prominent that everything in life triggers a negative response. Naturally, you will often lose your temper; you will have no control over your words. But if you begin to discipline yourself while you are young, this need not happen.

Controlling an emotion such as anger is a great art, one that you have to work at day by day. Learn to watch your mind and discipline yourself. Make a resolve, "I will not be like everybody else. As I grow, I will become more calm. I can have more control over my temper. I will not blow up over little things."

Do not allow yourself to be a slave to anger. If you overcome it, you will develop immense mental power. You cannot imagine the power that you will acquire, the peace that you will enjoy.

In the *Mahabharata*, grandfather Bhisma lay on a bed of arrows giving wonderful teachings to his family and friends, although his body was pierced everywhere by those sharp arrows. Even in that state, his mind was perfectly under control because he had always been such a disciplined personality. When his grandson Yudhishthira asked him for the secret of success in life, Bhisma said that the great secret of success is mastery over your speech.

Do not let your speech be harsh no matter what your situation. Do not excuse your defects. Mahatma Gandhi was able to do great works, yet nobody heard him shouting, nobody saw him in a state of anger.

When we are angry, we hurt ourselves and others in three ways: physically through our violent actions, vocally through our uncontrolled words, and mentally through our ill will. In the attempt to control your anger, the first step is to discipline your actions: do not express anger through your body by throwing things around or hitting people. You may not be able to stop yourself from saying angry things, but at least you are not being physically violent!

As you advance to the next stage of maturity, you do not need to say abusive things either; you have control over your speech. At this stage you may still be thinking angry thoughts, but at least you are not compelled to verbalize them.

When you reach the next stage, you have succeeded in controlling the mind also. And when you have controlled thoughts, words and actions, you have disciplined yourself perfectly and negative states such as anger are no longer a problem.

Control of anger is possible only if you do not allow yourself to harbor resentment within your heart. It is not enough just to hold back bitter words. If your heart is filled with bitterness, if you are silently thinking, "This boy has harmed me. I want to tell him to go to hell, but I won't say it! But all my life I'll remember how he harmed me," then your anger is sure to rear its head sooner or later.

If you are harboring internal resentment, your mental energy will be depleted. But by spiritual understanding you can learn to replace anger with true compassion for those who harm you. You develop sympathy for people who cannot control their evil actions, just as you have sympathy for people who have a cold or a cough.

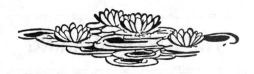

Thus, these ten important aspects of virtuous conduct that were taught by Sage Manu:

- **Dhriti**—Firmness
- **Kshama**—Forgiveness, Forbearance
- **Dama**—Control of the Senses
- **Asteya**—Nonstealing
- **Shaucha**—Purity of Body and Mind
- **Atma Vinigraha**—Control of the Mind
- **Dhee**—Purity of Intellect
- **Vidya**—Knowledge
- **Satya**—Truthfulness
- **Akrodha**—Absence of Anger

must be held as your ideal, and practised according to your capacity day by day. If you do so, then you are pursuing the path of *dharma*. And since you are pursuing the path of *dharma*, yours will be the victory! Not only will you have success in your practical life, but you will attain God-realization as well!

THE JOY OF SHARING

If you have a particular talent, you should be able to use it to help humanity. If you have wealth, you should be able to use it to do good deeds for others.

Generosity with whatever you possess, rather than selfishness, leads to true success. The moment you think, "Let me secure my own happiness, and let everyone else go to the dogs!" you actually shut the door to happiness. Miserliness leads to misery. Generosity leads to great joy and prosperity. The more you give the more you get.

The Smokey Buddha

In Tibet there are certain temples where there are a thousand statues of Buddha lined up, and when a worshipper comes, he chooses one particular statue to which to offer flowers and incense. Once there was a Buddhist monk who had come to worship in such a temple, and he had chosen as his Deity one of the thousand Buddhas.

Every day he brought butter-filled lamps, incense, and camphor, and he burned them before his particular Deity. Of course, whenever he did so, the fragrance wafted from his Deity and travelled to other Buddhas. Observing this, the monk thought, "All my money is being wasted for other Buddhas. My offerings should go only to my Buddha."

So he thought and thought about what he could do to correct the situation, and finally came up with the idea of creating a barrier. Then he brought some planks of wood and walled in his Buddha in such a way that the fragrance of the incense no longer travelled to the other statues.

Day by day, the monk watched the incense burn only for his Buddha and he was happy. But as time passed, he realized his great error: his Buddha became black from the confined smoke while all the other Buddhas remained bright and clean.

This story has a great message for you. If you do everything only for your little self, then the Buddha—the Self within you—becomes black. But when you share your knowledge and talents generously with others, you grow ever more bright and pure. When you are generous with others, nature continues to supply you with new resources, and new talents begin to unfold within your heart.

How did great personalities such as Mahatma Gandhi accomplish so much? How did they help so many other people? Humility and selflessness were their secrets.

Once a child came to Mahatma Gandhi and said, "Please tell me, why do people call you *Mahatma* or Great Soul?" And Mahatma Gandhi replied, "Because I am the littlest in this world."

The Scholar Who Pretended to be a Coolie

In Bengal there once lived a man named Ishwar Chandra, who was renowned for his many talents and great scholarship. Because of his abilities, "Vidyasagar"—which means "ocean of knowledge"— was added to his name and he was then known as Ishwar Chandra Vidyasagar.

Once this renowned scholar travelled by train to Calcutta, and when the train arrived at the station he saw an English lady standing there with a huge box. She started crying out, "Coolie! coolie!" hoping to find a man to carry it, but there was no coolie around.

Seeing her predicament, Ishwar Chandra said, "I am here to help you." Thinking he was a coolie, the lady gave him the big box and all her other things and he carried them to the *tanga*, a horse-driven carriage. When she sat down in the *tanga* she reached for her purse, intending to give him money. At that moment she realized that he was the famous Ishwar Chandra Vidyasagar.

As the story illustrates, doing humble or menial tasks for your own good or for the good of others does not mean you become lesser. Rather, whenever your ego becomes little, you become greater. Greatness lies in selflessness, in sharing yourself generously with others, in living to bring delight to others.

THE IMPORTANCE OF GOOD MANNERS

In the life of every individual, possessing good manners—known in Sanskrit as *sadachar* or *shishtachar*—is the foundation for good education and true progress.

On the simplest level of understanding, good manners refer to the rules of courtesy that you learn from childhood. For example, being disrespectful to your parents or elders is not good manners. To suddenly get up and start shouting whatever comes to your mind when you are seated in a group is not good manners. To reach for the dessert at the beginning of a meal instead of waiting for the right time is not good manners. To interrupt when someone is talking to you is not good manners.

The need for courtesy applies to all situations, at home, with your relatives, and with your peers. If your manners are good, you make yourself, as well as the people around you, more comfortable.

In this day and age, however, you are exposed to the values of television shows and movies. As a result, much of the language and manners you are exposed to do not reflect a spiritual sensitivity to the value of goodness and respect.

Further, even when you have been well-taught as a child, as you get older you may develop the erroneous idea that you should abandon the good manners you learned in childhood, thinking them to be out of fashion. One should always respect parents and elders. Unfortunately, in these modern times, giving such respect is considered old fashioned. This view is completely incorrect.

If you don't have good manners, then what you create is disharmony. Even a seemingly minor and unimportant act of bad manners can provoke disharmony. For example, there can be a hundred people seated in a hall and all is calm and quiet. Then one person gets up to leave and instead of closing the door softly, he or she lets it bang. Or, during a program, one person may decide to move across the room just to hand someone a slip of paper. Many little inconsiderate moves can create a disturbance. It may all seem very innocent, but you must realize that when you start doing something abnormal to draw the attention of others, you are pampering your ego—and that is ill-mannered.

Although being courteous is an expression of good manners, being overly courteous could become impractical. The following humorous episode reflects how it is possible to go too far in displaying good manners:

There were two grownup relatives who decided to take a trip by train. At the station when it was time to board, one gestured to the other, saying, "You first." and the other said, "No, no, no, you are far superior to me, so, after you." Well, this continued until they heard the train whistle and then begin to move on. Now that is not what is meant by good manners. That is overstepping the bounds of practicality, which good manners should not do.

Furthermore, good manners should enable you to practise concentration, control your senses, and have a certain degree of control over your moods and temper. Good manners also implies humility, mastery over speech, and the ability to handle all situations in an efficient way.

In the *Upanishadic* times when students were receiving their education, they were given a message: *"Matri devo bhava"*—"Let your mother be your God;" *"Pitri devo bhava"*—"Let your father be your God;" *"Acharya devo bhava"*—"Let your teacher be your God." The teaching went on to say that you should not conduct yourself in a harmful way, or in a way that is not in agreement with the scriptures. Whenever you are in doubt, reflect upon how great men conducted themselves in similar situations and follow their inspiring examples.

If you do not have good manners, then all your education becomes hollow. If you do have good manners, then you radiate harmony and peace. You can even deal with people who are rude and smooth out their rudeness. In other words, no matter what type of company you are in, good manners act to promote harmony and peace.

Going still deeper into this practice, *sadachar* means righteous conduct—a conduct that can lead you to *Sat*, which means Truth. *"Satyameva jayate naanritam."*—"Truth alone triumphs, not falsehood."

It is sincerity that is the foundation of righteousness. Always realize that you should be true to yourself, and on that basis you should be able to practise truth without developing fear or doubt. Your sincerity will ultimately win because truth triumphs no matter how difficult a situation may be.

Suffering and sacrificing for the sake of truth becomes a foundation for building tremendous willpower. On the other hand, it will not secure happiness to adopt insincere ways to overcome rough situations in life. Rather, your future will become dark.

The Yamas and Niyamas

In developing your standards for righteous conduct, always remember the great *yamas* and *niyamas* of Raja Yoga. The *yamas,* or ethical restraints, include *ahimsa* (nonviolence), *satyam* (thinking, speaking and acting on the basis of truthfulness), *brahmacharya* (control and sublimation of sex-energy), *asteya* (nonstealing—in both its gross and subtle forms), and *aparigraha* (noncovetousness or nonhoarding of possessions you do not need).

The *niyamas,* or ethical observances, include *shauch* (maintaining physical and mental purity), *santosh* (contentment), *tapas* (austerity), *swadhyaya* (the study of scriptures and repetition of *mantra*) and *Ishwar-pranidhan* (surrender to God).

The *yamas* are restraints. They refer to things you should not do: do not kill, do not hurt others, do not lie, do not steal, do not covet, etc. The *niyamas* are observances. They refer to things that you should do: you should elevate your mind by *satsanga* and study of scriptures, you should keep your body and mind pure and healthy, you should be able to practice contentment and surrender to God. All these *yamas* and *niyamas* are important ingredients of *sadachar*—the practice of righteous conduct.

There is a profound illustration from ancient times about the great hero Yudhishthira—a person with a very high standard for righteous conduct. Once his teacher gave Yudhishthira and his classmates the task of learning the *yamas*. When the teacher followed up on the assignment and asked the students if they had learned their lessons, they all said "yes" except Yudhishthira. He kept quiet.

The teacher then became extremely angry. "How is it that you could not learn such a simple lesson by heart?" he shouted. Again Yudhishthira kept quiet. Displeased, the teacher beat Yudhishthira black and blue with a stick (which was quite normal in those days) and although Yudhishthira was beaten, still he remained quiet.

Suddenly the teacher realized why Yudhishthira was silent. He was completely engrossed in examining his mind to see whether or not he had really learned the lesson of nonviolence. It is one thing, Yudhishthira reflected, to say that nonviolence is the highest virtue, but it is entirely another thing to practise it.

Similarly, if you read the story of Mahatma Gandhi and other great personalities of the world, you will find that *sadachar* was the foundation of their growth and progress. The greatest of all personalities were men of God-realization, men of spiritual knowledge. Their lives were founded on *sadachar*, and they became examples for others of how the lamp of righteousness can remove the barren darkness of life. Therefore, follow the path of *sadachar*, enrich your personality with Divine virtues, and attain God-realization.

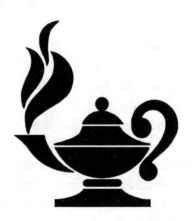

"VITAMINS & MINERALS" FOR MENTAL HEALTH

Just as the physical body depends upon vitamins and minerals for its health, the mind depends upon spiritual vitamins and minerals. These include:

Vit A: Aspiration, Adaptability, *Ahimsa* (nonviolence)

Vit B: Blissfulness, *Brahmacharya* (sex-restraint)

Vit C: Cheerfulness, Compassion

Vit D: Dispassion, Discrimination, Devotion

Vit E: Egolessness, Enquiry of "Who am I?"

Vit M: Meditation

Vit P: Persistent effort

The various Divine virtues, repetition of *mantra*, prayer, and acts of goodness are the minerals needed for promoting mental health. When you make use of these spiritual vitamins and minerals under the guidance of expert yogis and sages, you are bound to enjoy mental peace and spiritual health all your life.

LEARN TO COMMUNICATE EFFECTIVELY

Another great virtue that you must develop in your relationship with others is the art of listening. If you listen well to what others are saying, they will also listen to what you have to say. People talk to each other a lot, but generally they are not listening. Friends and relatives may chat and chat for hours, but there may be no real inner communication between them.

The Strange Conversation

Once there were two men who had been great friends when they were young, growing up together in the same village. Eventually, one became a merchant and moved away to another city and the other became a farmer and remained in the village. Separated geographically in this way, the two friends lost touch with each other.

Many years passed, and one day a message came to the farmer that his merchant friend was in the hospital in a nearby city. Eager to see his old friend, the farmer decided to go there for a visit.

However, the farmer, who was in his sixties, had become hard of hearing. So now, he thought to himself, "How can we talk to each other if I can't hear what he is saying?" In an attempt to solve the problem, he imagined what the conversation would be about and planned out his words and responses in advance:

"I will greet my friend and say, 'How are you?' And he will answer, 'Well, I am feeling fine.' Then I will say, 'Thank God you are feeling fine.' Then I will say, 'What did you eat for breakfast?'" In this way, the farmer planned the entire conversation in his mind.

Having rehearsed everything well, the farmer went to the hospital. Seeing the merchant he said, "Dear friend, it has been such a long time since I have seen you. How do you feel?"

"I am feeling miserable," replied the friend.

Unable to hear these words, the farmer said, "Thank God."

Hearing this response and not knowing that his friend was becoming deaf, the merchant thought with great annoyance, "He is seeing me again after such a long time, and he is happy that I am miserable! What type of friend is he?"

The farmer said, "What have you eaten today?"

The merchant replied in anger, "I've eaten poison."

"Well, good digestion!" said the farmer—and the merchant became all the more angry.

Then the farmer asked, "Who is your doctor?"

The angry merchant replied, "Death!"

"Oh," said the farmer, "he has a lucky foot. Wherever he goes, he succeeds."

By this time the merchant was so angry that he started shouting, and had the farmer thrown out.

This story gives an exaggerated example of lack of communication. But it humorously points out the nature of that problem and the need to avoid it.

In families, in schools, in the business world—wherever people must work together—many misunderstandings develop due to lack of real communication. When people talk to each other, they are involved in their own mental confusions and have difficulty really listening to one another. From morning to night, people go on talking about so many things, but often there is no real communication.

When there is no noise, you can hear even a leaf falling, but when there is a lot of noise, you cannot really hear anything at all. Similarly, if you learn how to relax and not let your ego overpower your mind, your communication with others improves and you become a good listener. But if your mind is filled with the noise of bitterness, anger, and hate, then you cannot hear what others are trying to tell you. It is in an atmosphere of love and harmony that people are able to really listen to each other.

4

YOU AND YOUR FAMILY

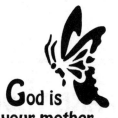

God is
in your mother,
in your father, in all.
When you give reverence to your elders,
God within them responds to you
with His Grace and helps you
meet the challenges
of your life.

PHILOSOPHICAL INSIGHT INTO FAMILY

It may seem that you just came to your parents from nowhere. But if you study the law of *karma* and reincarnation, you learn that you are an incarnating soul—not an individual body—and you come into a family on the basis of your previous *karma* (actions). Further, in the process of reincarnation, you have had hundreds and hundreds of families. Although in Western society these ideas are not generally understood, in the Hindu tradition they are ingrained from childhood.

After death the spirit, according to its *karmas*, chooses a family. You are actually the one who chooses the family to which you come. A little exercise of intellect is needed to understand that point.

If you had a strong musical inclination in your previous birth, you will now choose a family in which parents encourage you in music from childhood. Suppose in your previous birth you were inclined to worship, mysticism, meditation, yoga exercises, or other aspects of yoga *sadhana* (spiritual discipline). In this birth, you would be drawn into a family which would encourage you in this direction, where you would see your parents performing worship and practising meditation.

Therefore, it is important to understand that you are drawn to a family for a Divine reason. Similarly, your parents have come in contact with you because of their *karmas*. Their souls also need certain experiences from you. So when parents and children come together, it is not by accident.

The family is meant to help you attain God-realization. As an incarnating soul you have been a traveller who has come and gone through so many families. It is hard to believe how many thousands of fathers and mothers you have had! It is equally as hard to believe how many thousands of times you have been a parent, and how many thousands of children you have had! And this process of reincarnation will continue until you attain God-realization.

Knowing this, you should not develop a sense of dissatisfaction: "If I had been born in a different family, everything I wanted would have been given to me. I would have had wonderful toys. I would have had a wonderful car. I would have had lots of freedom. But alas, I have not been born into such a perfect family." Ideas like that should not enter your mind. You should not find fault with the family into which you belong, because that has been well arranged by a Divine plan to suit all the needs of your evolution.

REAL EDUCATION
BEGINS AT HOME

It is not just what you learn from schools that makes you educated. The greatest teachings are given in the family—not anywhere else. In schools and colleges you may get the most advanced technical instruction, but only from the family do you learn how to develop real character and integrity.

You may get the highest grades in school. You may be offered scholarships and receive numerous awards for excellent achievement. But if you do not know how to be in harmony with your parents, your brothers and sisters, or with your husband or wife, then you have learned very little. If you do not know the art of pleasing the people around you, then you have not received the real education that allows you to be more noble and integrated and to live a truly purposeful life.

In an ideal family, "ideal" does not imply that everybody in the family is a saint. What it implies is that an ideal of harmony is followed with great sincerity of purpose. Father and mother must strive to live in harmony with each other. Children must learn to be sympathetic to the problems of their parents, and parents to be sympathetic to the problems of the children. The older members of the family must be reverenced, and their wisdom must serve as a guiding light to the younger people. When people live together in such an ideal family, there is great joy.

This does not mean that there will always be good times for everyone in the family. Difficult times will come every now and then, but when you share adversity with the other members of your family, everyone receives healthy encouragement and learns how to move forward with greater wisdom and strength.

In an ideal Hindu home if someone becomes sick and the doctor tells him that he should not eat *rasgulas* or *pakoras* (sweets and savories), then the other family members will also forego eating these treats. This is symbolic of the fact that each family member must share in the difficulties of the others, which provides a healthy discipline and helps to foster joyous and caring relationships from which everyone learns the greatest lessons of life.

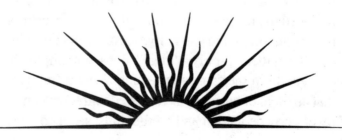

GIVE REVERENCE
TO YOUR ELDERS

In an ideal family there should be a special spiritual feeling about elderly family members. However, this special reverence is often absent in modern society. In many homes in the West, when parents become old they are removed from the family unit and taken to old age homes, leaving the family insecure and unstable.

In the traditional Hindu home, the family unit is often quite large. Father, mother, children, grand-parents, and other older people in the family all live together. The elders are not discarded, but reverenced, and their knowledge is enjoyed by all. This ideal should be kept in view.

The scriptures say that when you touch the feet of the elders and receive blessings from them, those blessings give you health, wealth, knowledge, peace, and prosperity. But when elders are discarded, you do not receive that blessing.

There is a humorous story that sheds light on the need to reverence one's elders:

A young married man in the West found his elderly father had become senile and a bother to himself and his wife. And so, he conversed about the problem with his wife, and they decided that since they did not have enough money to put him into an old age home, they must throw him off a bridge! So the man put his very thin, elderly father into a basket and carried him to a nearby bridge.

When he was just about to do the hideous deed, the father said, "Oh my son, when you throw me over the side, don't throw away the basket; take that home with you." And the son said, "Why, father, are you so concerned about the basket?" The father replied, "Because, my son, your son will need the basket someday for you!" Of course, these words touched the son's heart and brought him to his senses, and he brought his father back to the house.

The type of culture in which parents are thrown out of the house when they become old is a culture that is focused on pleasure. In such a culture, one's main concern is, "How much pleasure can I have? How much free time can I have?" And that culture is bringing a lot of misery in Western society. All the drug addiction, all the restless minds, all the stress, criminality, and perversion arise because family life is not healthy; it lacks ethical values. If you want a world with real peace and harmony, promoting a healthy family life is the secret.

HONOR YOUR PARENTS

The *Upanishad* says: *"Matri devo bhava"* —"Let your mother be God," and *"Pitri devo bhava"* —"Let your father be God." These words and the concept behind them lead to the development of a deeply reverential attitude between children and their parents.

According to the Hindu ideal, the first thing that children do when they first wake up in the morning is to go to their mother and father and touch their feet; in turn, the mother and father bless them. Even a grown up person will touch the feet of his father and his mother. Your mother may touch the feet of her mother-in-law.

What does this imply? It implies that you worship God in all those who are elders. In turn, when you receive blessings from a person, it is not the person's ego, but rather God within the person Who extends this grace to you.

The scriptures say that receiving blessings from the elders gives spiritual nourishment to your personality. You gain health, long life, bright intellect, and the moral basis to fight the battle of life in a heroic way. In turn, you help your mother and father to recognize that they are instruments of God. This mutual respect between children and their elders is a powerful cultural process.

Touching the feet of your parents has great merit even from a practical point of view. It sets up a psychological atmosphere of harmony. Suppose that your father is angry. If you touch his feet, see what happens to his anger. If your mother does not want to talk to you, practice a little bit of Hindu manners and touch her feet. Then wait quietly for an hour and try to speak to her again. She will be much more open-minded.

The moment you touch the feet of a person, that person becomes humble. Whatever their mood, they will bless you immediately, instinctively, whether they want to or not. The blessing comes from God deep within them. God is in your mother, in your father, in all. If you reverence a person, then the God within the person will respond to you and help you.

If you have made an error, you should not be proud or egoistic and cling to it. The moment you recognize an error, you should be able to ask for forgiveness from your parents or from whomever you have harmed. That builds strong character. When you admit your error, you show that you want to overcome it. Then, no matter what you have done, people look at you with greater love, and they become more tolerant and understanding.

You should learn the art of harmonizing with your parents. If you have a problem, learn to talk to your parents. Do not keep your problems hidden in your heart. Parents can advise you, help you, support you. In turn, you enhance the joy of your parents by your presence, by your growth and evolution. Through this mutual process, life becomes richer for all.

Growing up in this modern, technological world, you have the opportunity to learn much more than your parents about many things. Schools and colleges now impart a very high level of academic knowledge in many fields. Such scientific and technological advancement was not available for your parents when they were growing up.

Although you may feel proud at times that you know things that your parents do not know, at the same time, you should be humble. Why? Because your parents are a profoundly important support for you. Do you remember when there was a show or a parade and your father would lift you up on his shoulders so you could see things from above? Knowing that you could see much more than your father, you might develop a false sense of your own importance—forgetting that all the while you were supported by the shoulders of your father. Similarly, in whatever you are now learning you are supported by your parents. You are on their shoulders—and you should not forget that.

THE VALUE OF FAMILY DISCIPLINE

If you are not disciplined at an early age, you may later fall prey to numerous evils such as bad association, drugs, drinking, and manifold perversions of modern materialistic society. Life then becomes a curse.

If you are left "free" to do whatever you want, according to your whims, you become mentally disbalanced. You are truly free when you possess a clear mind and the ability to control your senses. Freedom comes when there is order and discipline, not when there is slavery to the senses.

When you are small, you might resent your parents for disciplining you. As you grow up, however, you appreciate them because of it. As you mature you understand that it was their responsibility to raise you well. You came into their lives as a tender stranger, and it was the duty of your parents to give you a sense of values, to train you, to educate you, to prepare you for bigger responsibilities in society and for higher purposes in life.

In the Hindu culture, the first stage in life is called *Brahmacharya Ashrama*, the disciplinary level. The more you allow yourself to be disciplined, the better and more joyous your life will be as time goes on. But if you are not disciplined from the early stages of your life, your future will be in turmoil. That discipline implies many things: discipline of the senses, of the mind, of the intellect, of the body.

The next stage of life is called *Grihastha Ashrama*—householder's life. When you enter into a householder's life, your purpose is not pleasure and fun—although these are an important part of life. The real purpose is to become a responsible person who can love another human being on a very profound level. Such profound love develops when husband and wife work together, help each other, sacrifice for each other. As children come into the family, that love begins to grow more and more if the family is living in an ideal way.

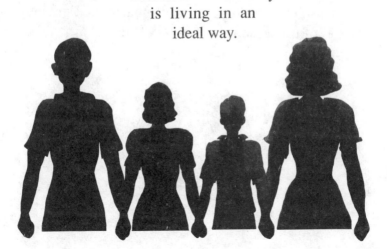

Married life is not a simple project. Fairy tales often end with the words: "then they were married and lived happily ever after." In the real world, however, this is not usually so. For many couples, the marriage ceremony is the entry into an intense battle of life!

Therefore, as you grow up, think deeply about the responsibilities involved in raising a family, and also the great role of the family in society. The ultimate goal of religion and spiritual philosophy is to make you selfless. When you enter into family life, you begin to learn humility. You begin to learn how to control your temper, to handle your disappointments. When you are alone it is very difficult to develop those virtues. But when you enter into a special relationship with your spouse and your children with the right attitude, you begin to develop spiritual maturity. Therefore, the householder's life is designed for more enrichment of your personality, more integration, more discipline. This discipline endows you with great mental strength and is of immense value for your spiritual growth.

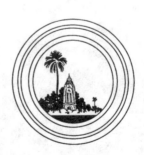

WHEN THE WORLD BECOMES YOUR FAMILY

In the Hindu tradition, the third stage in one's life (after *Brahmacharya Ashrama* and *Grihastha Ashrama*) is *Vanaprastha Ashrama,* or retired life. In ancient times when people retired, they went to the forest and they practised more austerity, more meditation, and lived a more religious life. There in the forest they set up schools so that they could share their experience with others as teachers.

Today the same ideal must be respected. Do not start dreaming of retiring one day from all work and buying a house in a city like Miami Beach so that you can do nothing but sit on a rocking chair and watch the travellers pass by. Rather, you must cherish the idea of always being bright and alert, of always possessing a mind that continues advancing.

Yoga teaches you that the mind is not the same as the brain or nervous system. It is beyond. The mind has a special Divine power that enables it to become stronger and more alert as you grow older and continue to discipline yourself. On the other hand, if you live your life in a haphazard fashion, without discipline and proper guidance, then as you age your mind becomes weak, and senility overtakes you. But if you are living properly, the older you become the brighter your mind becomes.

So *vanaprasta* life is a life of intense service to society in which you utilize and share all that you have learned through the disciplined childhood years of *brahmacharya* and the profound experiences of *grihastha* or family life. The highest level reached in this process is *sanyasa,* or renunciation, which is the fourth stage.

Renunciation implies that a person belongs to all of humanity. He does not claim any home as his own or any family as his own. His sole purpose is to love God and share that love with all of humanity.

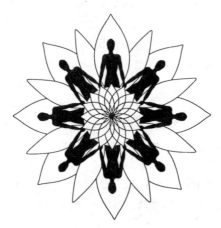

THE DIRECT PATH TO RENUNCIATION

If you have developed a profound interest in spiritual life and have already attained great *vairagya,* or dispassion, you may adopt *sanyasa,* or renunciation, without entering into *grihastha* (householder) or *vanaprastha* (retired) stages of life. In a healthy and mature way, you may choose to remain a *brahmachari* (a celibate) throughout your life. In doing so, you are referred to as a *naishthika brahmachari*—one who has taken the vow of *brahmacharya* for his whole life.

If, as a *brahmachari* student, due to very advanced impressions, or *shubha samskaras,* you are able to transmute the urge for pleasure into an urge for Liberation and go directly into *sanyasa*, your parents need not be upset nor view this as something tragic. It is due to very good *karma* from the past. However, with the help of your parents you should look deeply into your mind to determine if you are choosing *sanyasa* because of some frustration or immaturity. If so, it would be wise for you to reconsider, because you will not succeed.

Adopting *sanyasa* should stem from full confidence within you. If you do not have that powerful urge, you will go astray in the name of *brahmacharya*. The path of *sanyasa* requires a resolute march on a heroic path and it should not be adopted on the basis of a shallow sentiment. The strength to make this choice belongs to only a small number who have developed great aspiration for Self-realization.

It requires a tremendous power to step beyond the biological urge which has chased the soul from life to life. But with the power of *vairagya* a person may step beyond it and allow himself to be disciplined by a spiritual teacher until passion is completely transmuted into *ojas shakti* (spiritual energy)—and that is the goal. Whether you are a *brahmachari* or a *grihasthi*, the goal is to realize, during this very life, that you are not a physical body.

Bhishma in the *Mahabharata* is an example of a *naishthika brahmachari*. Because of his mastery over his senses, he had developed the psychic power of controlling his death at his will. Some great personalities such as Sri Shankaracharya embraced *sanyasa* without ever entering into householder life. These enlightened personalities have no need to follow the ancient plan of *ashramas* (stages in life). They are enlightened souls who began with *brahmacharya* and through *brahmacharya* attained *Brahman*—the goal of life.

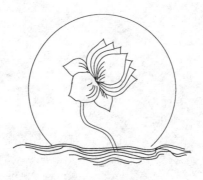

A family that nurtures the physical, mental and spiritual health of its members is indeed a blessing! Without the peace and security that is nurtured by a healthy family life, it is difficult to unfold the deeper qualities of the soul. If you live without hope, harmony, or adaptability at home, you grow up to be a discontented and distracted person. As such, there is very little good that you can do for yourself or for society.

The concept of an ideal family which we have been describing in these pages is important not only for Hindus, but for all human beings everywhere in the world. It is the foundation for developing the inner peace and fulfillment that gives meaning to life.

May God bless you with a family that encourages you to live with discipline, with love, and with respect for all of creation. And as you mature may you learn to serve the whole world as your family, and through loving service attain God-realization!

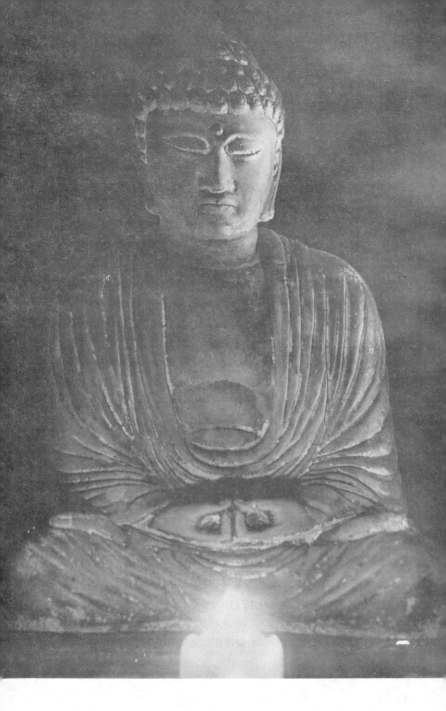

Lord Buddha

5

FACING THE CHALLENGES
OF TODAY'S WORLD

It is your
birthright to vibrate
with strength and courage.
Nothing is impossible for you.
The spirit that rules the earth
and the heavens is the
indweller of your
heart!

THE ILLUSION OF SEXUAL "FREEDOM"

There is a great misconception in today's world. Members of the modern generation feel that they are more culturally advanced than people who have come before them because they enjoy more sexual freedom than their forefathers did. They consider this so-called freedom as a mark of progress—as something highly desirable. But the truth is actually quite different.

Unbridled passion and uncontrolled sexuality existed in the past just as it does now, but in olden times it was looked down upon by society. It was viewed as a taint of personality which an individual should not be proud of. An individual who was a prey to weaknesses was advised to seek the guidance of the wise. In the past, weaknesses in character were not adored nor sanctioned.

But today people have started worshipping their lower selves. They are proud of sexual freedom. They are not ashamed of living lives of slavery to the senses. Young people in this materialistic society are led by the communications media and by the misguided example of many of their elders to believe that sex is fun and that fun is what life is all about.

They are not aware of the fact that by their so-called sexual freedom they are degrading themselves physically, psychologically, and morally, and in addition they are contributing to the degradation of society. Any promiscuity and frivolous sex-involvement leads to a debilitated mind, ill health, and a guilty conscience.

Anyone, regardless of age or stage of life, who is eager to attain Self-realization must not permit himself to be tempted by the lures of sex. If he submits himself to gross pleasures with the notion that later he will overcome them, he is terribly wrong. He becomes like a person who has placed his feet in quicksand—no matter how much he tries to free himself, he continues to sink deeper and deeper into illusions.

Thus, *grihasthas* (householders) and their children must deeply understand that in order to be truly successful, happy and fulfilled in life, they must reverence the human body and recognize the profound nature of the sex relationship. And ultimately, as they mature, their minds must eventually outgrow or outstep the illusion of sex altogether.

The mind that does not evolve beyond illusions of pleasure—and sex-pleasure is one of the most powerful of those illusions—carries those illusions into old age and even beyond! Thus you see many people who are in their seventies or eighties who are still imprisoned by those illusions. And the spirit moves from one body to another body, incarnation after incarnation, pursuing them.

A pleasure-loving person who runs from one mate to another until he is 90 years old is not really successful or happy. He is in a most miserable situation. But, once you begin to overcome that illusion, tremendous power is released within you and all great virtuous qualities begin to unfold in your personality.

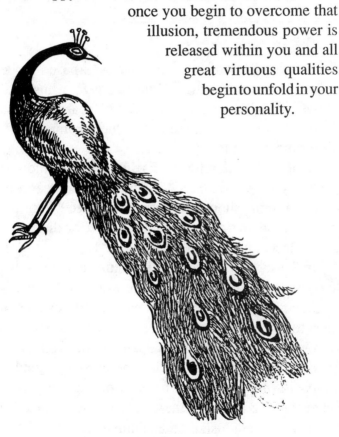

WHAT IS BRAHMACHARYA?

The youth of today are constantly exposed to the charms of materialistic culture through films, TV shows, and radio programs. It is for this reason that the ideal of *Brahmacharya* seems like such an impossibility for most people.

Brahmacharya refers to discipline of the amorous part of your personality—discipline in the realm of sex. Your mind should not become obsessed with sex. In these modern times, this topic needs to be discussed and reflected upon with great sincerity.

In this modern, materialistic culture, it appears that to be more sensuous is to be more wonderful. If a boy or girl is always going out on dates, they are considered most fortunate. But that is not so in the Hindu culture, which considers such preoccupation with dating as a break in *brahmacharya*. This is so because your mind—which is supposed to be focused on studying your school lessons as well as the scriptures—is involved in fancies and the illusion of attachments.

When you begin to date at a young age, fancies develop in your mind. You begin to admire people just for their looks and other superficial aspects of the personality. You may feel you have fallen in love, when really you know very little about love.

When you become infatuated with a person you have dated, and feel that he or she is the perfect person for you, what you should ask yourself is, "What would happen to me if I were to live with that person for a long time—not just date him or her for a month or two?"

There are two ways you can seek the company of the opposite sex: one is on the plane of human friendship, and the other is when you are seeking a partner in a relationship. In the first case, you spend recreational time with others, you study with them. There is no harm in such human companionship and it plays an important part in growing up.

In the second case, when you are going out with the intention of seeking a partner, you should be careful. Be sure you know a great deal about the person before you get entangled, before you decide that you have found the one you want to marry.

Living in the West, a Hindu young man or woman has the opportunity to go out with an American young man or woman, and as a result can become seriously involved with that person. In such a situation, you must ask yourself what you want your married family life to be like. Do you want your children to be brought up according to Hindu culture, or Christian culture, or

Jewish culture—or no religious culture at all? You must think of the many implications of your relationship with that partner as time passes by; you must understand all the consequences and all the psychological adjustments you will have to make.

Often what appears wonderful in a superficial relationship is not really so. There is a humorous story that points this out:

Once upon a time a prince was passing through a village on his horse when he suddenly saw a young girl. She was so beautiful that he immediately fell in love with her. He got right off his horse and went over to her and said, "I am a prince and I am going to marry you."

The girl, who was a farmer's daughter, was mature-minded and she realized that she would not be happy with the prince. She also realized that the prince was going after her just because of his wild fancies. So she said to him, "Let me think about it."

"There is no thinking about it," he said. "I am a prince and what I command must be obeyed." And she replied, "All right, I will prepare to become your bride. Come in three days."

Overjoyed with his expectations, the prince left the village. Immediately, the wise girl took a strong potion and created such havoc within her body that she looked ghastly. So when the prince returned and saw her he said, "Where is that beautiful girl?" "Here I am!", she replied. Because all he was interested in was her physicalappearance, the prince became terribly disillusioned, and with disgust he jumped on his horse and took off, losing all interest.

There is so much illusion involved when you try to find someone to marry. Therefore, it is greatly advisable that you make friends with your parents and learn from their judgement.

In western society, children know that when they grow to be a certain age, legally they are free to make their own decisions. But that freedom means nothing. Real freedom comes when you can organize and handle your life with a clear mind. Just being legally free puts you in a strange and confused world.

So don't be deluded by the letter of the law when you reach the time when you are thinking of marriage. Learn to communicate with your parents. When you feel that you are mature enough to have a marriage partner, and you have someone in mind, introduce that person to your parents, talk to your parents, and then think about what they have to say. Reflect on the situation a hundred times before you get into it. If you don't, terrible problems may develop. If you don't believe this, just study the statistics on marriage in the West. There are so many householders whose marital problems lead to great emptiness and eventual divorce.

Whether you are married or not, being a sensuous person is not your goal. You have to control the senses. Householder's life, or *Grihastha Ashrama*, is really an extension of *Brahmacharya Ashrama*.

In the disciplinary stage, *brahmacharya* was confined only to your body—keeping your body pure. In the *Grihastha Ashrama* stage you begin to understand that *brahmacharya* must include discipline of the mind as well.

When you are married, you should maintain sexual fidelity to your husband or wife. This requires discipline and depth of understanding. Through sexuality, you bring forth children and then help to educate them in all aspects of practical and spiritual life. This is a great responsibility. The sexual relationship is never meant just for fun.

As householders mature, they rise beyond the sexual demand of the body and develop *brahmacharya* to a still higher level. By the time you have perfected your *grihastha* responsibilities, you are ready, according to Hindu tradition, to retire and enter into *vanaprastha*, a stage in which you eventually become an absolute *brahmachari*—physically, mentally, and intellectually. In the highest *brahmacharya*, your intellect flows constantly toward God. *Brahmacharya* literally means living and moving in *Brahman*.

In its early stage, then, the practice of *brahmacharya* begins with the discipline of the sexual aspect of your personality. That sexual aspect can be the most dominating aspect in one's personality and if it is not taken care of, then all one's senses go astray. On the other hand, if you practise *brahmacharya* in the right sense, you develop what is referred to as *ojas shakti* (spiritual energy). *Ojas shakti* gives you a personal magnetism, a magnetism that comes from your spiritual personality and endows you with special power and energy.

It was that type of *brahmacharya* that was the secret of all great persons. It was the *brahmacharya* of Hanuman that enabled him to cross the ocean. It was the *brahmacharya* of Swami Vivekananda that made him such a powerful personality that just a few of his words impressed thousands of people. It was the *brahmacharya* of Mahatma Gandhi that made him lead his country to freedom. It was the *brahmacharya* of Jesus that led him to heights of spiritual glory.

Brahmacharya gives you an amazing mental power because you are not losing your mental energy over the demand of senses. Your mind understands, "The real me is spirit, beyond sexes." With this understanding you rise beyond multiple illusions.

The study of *brahmacharya* is a profound study not to be found in the western world. Strangely enough, western religious systems have not probed deeply into it. But in the Indian culture, *brahmacharya* is considered of utmost importance.

The scriptures say, *"Brahmacharyena tapasa devo mrityum-upaaghnata."* —"By *brahmacharya* and austerity Gods attained victory over death." You too are essentially Divine, and as you practise *brahmacharya* and austerity, you too can become free of death, and realize that you are the imperishable Absolute Self!

KEEP YOUR SPIRITS HIGH

It is your birthright to vibrate with strength and courage, to face life like a hero, to take things in stride with a happy heart. Until you become Enlightened, however, you are bound to become depressed about your problems from time to time. The idea that you can be happy and cheerful at every moment is unrealistic. The mind will always have its ups and downs. When the clouds of dejection do enter your mind, you can drive them away by adopting the following techniques:

• Practise hatha yoga and *pranayama* (breathing) exercises whenever you feel your spirit beginning to sink. These exercises bring harmony and balance to the mind and body. Or you may want to swim or jog or go for an invigorating walk in a beautiful natural setting. Just changing the atmosphere so that you can relax often causes your depressed mood to give way to a cheerful one.

• Do not take too seriously the negative thoughts that invade your mind when you are depressed. These thoughts are baseless. When you are dejected, you tend to imagine every terrible thing possible about yourself and become steeped in self-pity. As your mind regains its strength, these thoughts will disappear.

• Always remind yourself that "All things pass away." View your dejection as a passing dark cloud and learn to wait and watch with patience. This strengthens your will and makes your personality very dynamic.

• Understand that adversity is a great teacher with a Divine purpose. If you face adversity with the right attitude, it helps you to overhaul your personality by bringing the things that are hidden in your unconscious to the surface. When you are strong enough, nature has a mysterious way of presenting you with the challenging situations that are needed for your evolution. Through each difficult situation, nature is as if whispering, "Can I tell you a secret? It's going to be a little painful, but you need to hear it!"

• When nature brings you these challenging eye-openers, do not be ungrateful. Do not let depression take over and rob you of time and energy. Rather, learn to quickly push away the dark clouds that gather in your mind by keeping busy and continuing to perform your duties.

Although some tasks may require a cheerful, clear mind, there are other tasks that you can perform even when the mind is more clouded. If the demands of your life in school, at work or at home do not allow you to alter your activity according to your moods, do not become upset. With patience and perseverance, you can gradually train yourself to fulfill all your responsibilities even in the most distressing of situations.

If you are a student and you have a term paper due, you cannot allow yourself to linger in dejection and say, "Until this mood goes, I cannot write. I am not inspired." Rather, train yourself well and you will eventually be able to turn in your assignments on time—no matter what!

• Learn the art of promoting a positive mind by performing good *karmas* (actions). If you want to be happy, do not cause unhappiness in others. Having consideration for others and serving them with a generous heart will bring you joy and contentment, and help you to be unaffected by the adversities of life.

• When everything seems wonderful and all your expectations are being fulfilled, don't let your mind get carried away by the feeling of elation. If you rejoice too much during prosperity, you are bound to become disappointed when the tide turns towards adversity.

• Above all, do not consider depression as a terrible problem and thus start becoming depressed about depression! Sometimes you must accept the fact that you are slightly lower in spirit. When an athlete has to jump a great height, he lowers his knees in preparation for the jump. Lowering is not always bad. Your depression is a temporary lowering of the spirit so that you can eventually jump a higher distance in spiritual understanding.

• Follow the example of great men and women, and do not allow yourself to become depressed over trifles. Rather, if you must be depressed, be depressed about the fact that you are still unenlightened, that you have not yet discovered the blissful presence of God within your heart.

If depression is due to the soul's longing to understand the profound secrets of life, and because of it you seek the answers that can lead you to the highest goals, then that depression is a great blessing in disguise. This is exemplified by Arjuna's dejection in the first chapter of the *Gita*. When Lord Krishna sees Arjuna's state, He is delighted because He knows that his disciple is now ready to receive the highest teachings. When your depression is based upon a deep urge to confront your illusions, like Arjuna, you become a true aspirant on the spiritual path and gradually discover immense spiritual strength.

Once you develop a deep-rooted understanding that you are the immortal Divine Self, the embodiment

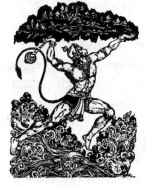

of bliss, you realize how ridiculous it is to enter into a state of dejection even for a moment. It is your birthright to vibrate with strength and courage. Nothing is impossible for you. The Spirit that rules the earth and the heavens is the indweller of your heart!

DON'T FALL PREY TO DRUGS

The message of Yoga or Vedanta philosophy is simply, "Do not fall prey to the lure of drugs." Drugs may seem to promise you mind-expanding, psychedelic experiences, or a sense of power and enhanced energy, or a feeling of confidence, sociability and well-being, or an escape from the problems of daily life, or even just enhanced concentration. However, all these promises, when viewed in the light of reason, are false. Instead of building your dreams on such empty promises, try to unfold the creative force of your own spirit by discovering your own inherent physical, mental and intellectual potential.

As you study the philosophy of Vedanta under proper guidance, you will understand the simple fact that any form of experience or realization produced by an external agency cannot lead to life's real attainments. Rather, it limits the unfoldment of your true potential, and restricts your possibility of experiencing what is really higher and more sublime in life.

In the 1960's and 1970's, many drug users adopted terms from oriental mysticism—be it Tibetan or

Vedantic—to justify the use of psychedelic drugs. For the most part, however, these terms were adopted without a true understanding of their philosophical meaning and importance. Life cannot be lived by empty words, no matter how grand or Divine their meanings may be.

Deluded by a weak will and a complexed mind, many drug users deceive themselves into believing that they are approaching Nirvana or Liberation, while in actuality they are moving away from that state of perfection towards its remotest shadows. No drug or outward prop can induce the sublime expansion of authentic spiritual experience.

Mental "Disconnectedness" Is Not Superconsciousness

The mind is actually a mystic energy which uses the brain and nervous system as the medium for its functions. The mind can be led to disconnect itself from the nervous system, or it can transcend it through the heights of spiritual consciousness.

Although both of these experiences are uniquely different from any known experience in the world, they are radically different from each other. Just as plus four and minus four are numerically alike, yet totally different in value, so too, the sublime experiences acquired through personality integration and meditation are totally different from the experiences revealed under the influence of drugs.

Every night in a natural way, one disconnects oneself from the conscious functions of the mind during sleep. Dreams manifest when the functions of the mind are not able to correlate with the grooves of the brain, and depending upon the intensity of the disconnection, one has diverse dream experiences.

The same phenomenon applies to the experiences artificially produced by psychedelic drugs. When the nervous system is suppressed by the force of a drug, the mind disconnects itself from it, resulting in psychedelic experiences. Lacking true insight, a drug user may consider this form of mental disconnectedness as the culmination of his mystic meditations. But in reality it is only a negative reflection of super-consciousness—beckoning him towards doom and darkness.

True mental expansion is experienced through the practice of concentration, meditation and *samadhi* (profound meditation). Concentration is the focusing of the mental energy on a point; it is a state of clarity in which the mind concentrates its energies without tension on one particular subject at a given time. Meditation is a still higher state of mind, one in which there is less effort involved in directing the mental energies to one point. In meditation, the mind flows on with greater placidity and serenity.

When the mind continues to be peaceful and tranquil, it enables one to behold the nature of the essential Self which is universal and eternal. It enables one to rise above the ego-center, and thereby to glimpse the glory of universal life. This is termed as *samadhi*.

This *samadhi* experience, which can arise only in a pure mind, does not conflict with the day-to-day world. On the contrary, it endows one with patience in confronting problems, faith in fighting the battles of life, perseverance in one's efforts, and depth of feeling in human relations. In short, this experience intensifies all that is noble in the human personality.

See Drug Abuse for What It Is

Drug-induced experiences are unable to broaden one's capacity for facing the realities of life with maturity and wisdom. Rather, these experiences hide within them the seeds of unresolved problems, and by hiding problems you can never solve them.

A user of drugs tends to become an escapist, veiling the voices of his conscience. He is, therefore, unable to understand the difference between the real and the ideal. If he becomes burdened by a brain and nervous system that have suffered irreversible damage, he is unable to harmonize his life in the plane of day-to-day reality and to create the proper circumstances for mental and spiritual expansion.

A person following a healthy, positive life may lack the effervescent experiences of "expansion" and "ecstasy" that he thinks the drug user enjoys, and due to delusion, he may think he is missing something. But this is a great error. The mind weakened by drugs and alcohol is a diseased mind, and not at all desirable. Such a mind is an insult to all that is good and sublime in humanity.

A MESSAGE TO HINDU STUDENTS LIVING IN THE WEST

As you mingle with young people in the West, and begin to follow their philosophy and their ways, your parents become frightened that you will become irreligious, that you will loose your Indian culture. Growing in the West gives you the possibility of a great deal of bad association through the constant exposure to TV and its programs, through people around who are becoming more and more materialistic. And it is indeed important to reflect upon this question: How can you sustain the profundity of Eastern culture in a Western world that is overpowered by materialism?

To help answer this question, religion must be understood from a broader point of view. Religion is not dress, it is not language, it is not external style—it is how you attune yourself with God in whatever setup or situation you are placed in. To be truly religious implies to develop an integrated personality that allows you to unfold the greatness of your potential. Can you, as Hindu young people growing up in the West, blossom into such integrated personalities?

Blending the Best of East and West

In Western culture, blind materialism, lack of human values, perversions involving drug abuse and rampant crime, as well as many other social ills are weighing heavily on society. These unhealthy elements of Western culture must be carefully avoided by you. However, the dynamic self-effort of the people, the orderliness, the rationality, and the scientific way of looking at things must be imbibed.

Much of India is burdened by the psychology of *tamas*, or inertia. The people have the most marvelous scriptures but they do not explore them. They allow themselves to feel sustained by the old glory of their culture, without making their culture ever new and vibrant.

Too many people in India are burdened by a sense of inactivity or inertia in their practical lives as well. The moment such people encounter a little frustration in their businesses, they will begin to quote the *Mahabharata*, assert that all of life is determined by

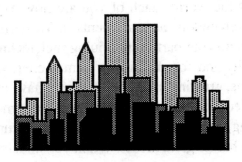

karmas, declare that money does not bring anything of value into life—and immediately resign themselves to inactivity! In the West people will not do so. The moment they fail in business they will go to a supermarket and get a job as a clerk, or do something else that will lift them out of their predicament as quickly as possible.

In Eastern culture time does not matter. God is eternal! If a lecture has been set for the early morning, those attending may not arrive until 9:00 or 10:00 o'clock or even until evening! In Western culture there is much more appreciation for the value of time, for punctuality.

In the Eastern culture, coordination of people in work that requires intense cooperation is lacking. Contrariwise, Western culture has given us many excellent examples of highly coordinated work. For example, see how spacecraft are developed and sent on their missions. See how hundreds of people put their minds and all their technical abilities together, and coordinate to accomplish dazzling tasks before the eyes of the world. Each of you are now exposed to those tremendous advancements in Western culture, and can do your part in continuing such technological creativity and coordination of human energy.

Thus, growing up in the West, you have to discard the defects of both the Eastern and Western ways of thinking, and assimilate the best of both cultures. Each culture has its great merits. When you understand and cherish Indian philosophy with a scientifically-oriented mind, you can present that philosophy in a better light to all of humanity.

The Blind and the Lame

This predicament of Eastern and Western cultures is just like the story of the lame man and the blind man. Perhaps you know that story:

The lame man lived miserably in one home and the blind man lived miserably in another. But one day they decided to work together. The lame man, who lacked useful legs, would climb on the shoulders of the blind man, who lacked useful eyes. As they walked in this fashion, the lame man used his good eyes to direct the blind man and show him the way.

When they came together, each helped the other. When they were apart, they could not help each other, nor were they helpful to themselves either.

The material culture of the West in itself is blind—it has no goal—and the Eastern culture in itself is lame—it has no legs. Oriental philosophy must climb on the shoulders of Western culture and show Westerners where their energy and technology should be directed.

Without that spiritual direction, the technological advancement of the West may lead to a tremendous calamity. It is already doing so. Young people as well as adults are becoming more and more perverted due to too much exposure to the TV, and too much comfort and laziness. Comfort has become identical with happiness. But in reality it is not so. Too much comfort has actually deprived people of the joy of life, and has thrown them into a stream of tension and stress in which they are drowning.

People have very little regard for themselves. Now a student does not depend on his own brain. He will not calculate unless he has a calculator. In the name of ease, people have discarded the sense of their own ability, and they now sit in front of machines with great awe and consider themselves lesser. That feeling has developed in the absence of spiritual culture.

If the West continues moving as it is, it will be like a blind man moving headlong into degradation and destruction. If the East remains isolated and enclosed within itself, and fails to share and imbibe the technological knowledge and skills of the West, it will be like the lame man. There will be no progress. Therefore, you young people and your parents living in the West have a unique opportunity to enjoy the best of both cultures, and blend them in your lives in a way that brings renewed health to both.

Become a Source of Inspiration
for Yourself and Others

Do not go after restless things such as drugs and bad company for your relaxation; go after *japa* (repetition of a Divine name or *mantra*), meditation, and hatha yoga exercises. These are the best reducers of stress in the body and the mind.

Become a source of inspiration to others. As an Indian who has assimilated both cultures—East and West—you are in a position to help humanity in the best way possible. You are also in the best position to explore within yourself the rich dimensions of your spirit.

Inspire your parents, teachers and the adults in your community to develop educational systems, schools, and colleges in which the two cultures can be well-blended.

The Eastern culture gives its treasure of philosophy and psychology. All the knowledge contained in the Vedas, the Upanishads and all the Vedic scriptures gives you the best solutions to the problems that humanity faces today. As a young person growing up in the West, you can disseminate that knowledge.

You, who have both cultures—the heritage and blessing of India as well as an education in the environment of the West—are in a position to do amazing things. From amongst you, great people like Swami Vivekananda, Mahatma Gandhi, and others, will arise, not from India, but from right here in Florida, or Pennsylvania, or New Jersey, or Ohio, or Texas, or somewhere else in the West!

Only where the two cultures blend will there be victory. Where there is a blending of the spirit of India and the self-effort of the West, where there is a blending of vision and action, where there are Krishna and Arjuna together, there there will be victory.

Krishna, with His Divine intellect, represents Indian philosophy, and Arjuna, with all his bows and arrows and weapons, represents all the technological advancement of the West. Where Krishna and Arjuna are together, there lies all the progress, all the victory. Keep this in view always as you strive for success and happiness.

Each of you is like a mighty river into which two streams of culture are flowing. May God bless you with the wisdom to extract the best from both and blend them into a healthy, radiant life. And may He lead you to the ultimate victory— the Ocean of Self-realization!

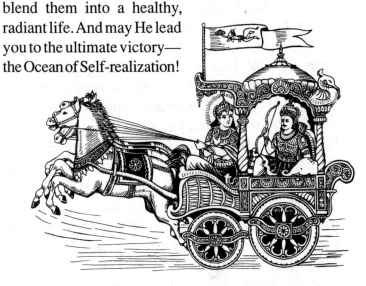

6

TOWARDS RADIANT HEALTH

Health of
the body and the mind
is the basis of prosperity, success,
ethical development, spiritual unfoldment,
radiant beauty and blessedness.
With health, the world becomes
a surging ocean of joy!

HATHA YOGA EXERCISES

What Is Hatha Yoga?

Hatha yoga is the world's most ancient system of physical and mental culture and it has been practised by yogis in India for centuries. It is a marvelous system of psychophysical exercises. The poses *(asanas)* of hatha yoga are performed with mental serenity as well as physical poise and grace. They are meant to promote elasticity of the spine and health of the nervous system. Yoga exercises nourish the roots of the nerves with subtle *prana* or vital energy and are, therefore, different from most systems of physical culture.

With the key of hatha yoga, you can unlock the infinite treasure of *prana*, regain lost health, acquire strength of mind, unfold hidden powers of the spirit, amass the wealth of willpower, attain success in every walk of life, and ascend to the mansion of Self-realization!

6

Bending your arms a
the elbows, bring the body
down so that the forehead
the chest, the two palms, the
two knees, and the two fee
are touching the ground. Only
these eight parts of the body
should touch the ground. This
is known as Sashtanga
Namaskara, or adoration
with the help of eight limbs
This is the complete act of
physical prostration. Slowly
breathe out.

5

4

Throw your left leg backwards.
The head, trunk and two legs will be
in a straight line. The whole body is
now supported by the palms of the
hands and the toes. Retain the breath.

3

Resting the palms of your hands on the ground alongside
your feet, throw your right leg backwards, while at the same time
bending the left knee. Your left knee is placed between the arms.
Raise your head and look above to the beautiful sky or the
effulgent Sun, or gaze at the ceiling above. Inhale slowly during
this process.

In a great swinging arc, bring your arms
forward and downward, keeping the elbows
straight, while bending your body at the waist
and trying to touch your toes with your fingers.
Slowly exhale during this process, and bring
your head down trying to touch your knees.

2

The
Poses
of
Surya
Namaskar

Inhale deeply while you stretch
your arms up above your head, moving
your gaze upwards and slightly bending
your head backwards.

1

Stand erect
with a majestic gait.
Fold your hands in
a prayerful manner.
The folding of the
hands is an ex-
pression of rever-
ence and adoration
to God, Who shines
in the sun.

Salutation

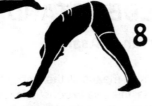

7

Breathing in, slowly raise the head like the raising of the hood of a snake. Bend the spine as you straighten the elbows. Behold the glory of the sky, turning the face upwards. This pose is similar to Cobra Pose or Bhujangasana.

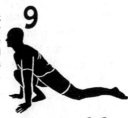

8

Exhaling, swing the trunk upwards and backwards, moving your head down, palms resting on the ground and the heels also firmly planted on the ground. The whole body appears to have a curvature like an inverted U.

9

Bringing the right leg forwards, assume a position symmetrical to that described in Pose 4. Inhale slowly.

10

These twelve poses constitute one cycle of Salutation to the Sun, or Surya Namaskar. Four complete cycles should be performed slowly and gracefully and one cycle should be performed in a very quick succession of the twelve poses.

The number of times that Surya Namaskar may be repeated can gradually be increased according to your strength and capacity.

Bring the left leg forward again and assume the same position as described in the Pose 3. Exhale slowly.

11

Stand as in Pose 2, with arms stretched out over your head and with the body bent backwards. Slowly breathe in.

12

Bring the hands down to your sides, again erect with a majestic gait, ready to repeat the next cycle of Surya Namaskar all over again.

to the Sun

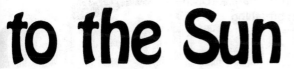

SHOULDER STAND
(Sarvanga Asana)

"Sarvanga" in Sanskrit means all the limbs of the body. So, as the name suggests, this *asana* benefits all parts of the body. It is an excellent posture for nourishing the blood and the nerves. It also has a particularly good influence in promoting the secretions of the thyroid gland, thereby assisting in healthy blood circulation, respiration, digestion, and genito-urinary function. This wonderful exercise promotes great health and vitality and should be practised every day.

Method

1. Lie flat on your back and relax your entire body.

2. Slowly lift your legs, bend your knees, and roll the hips over the shoulders.

3. Continue to lift the trunk, hips, and legs until they are vertically aligned. In the same movement, with the elbows on the floor close to the body, raise the forearms and support the back at the waist with the palms of the hands. Keep the body steady so that the chin presses firmly into the chest. The whole weight of the body now rests on the shoulders and elbows.

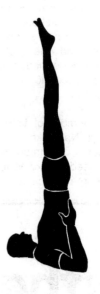

Breathe normally. You may also practise repetition of *mantra* (Divine name) along with breathing.

PLOW POSE
(Hala Asana)

This *asana* appears like a farmer's plow or *hala* when performed. Therefore, it is called Hala Asana (plow pose). With this *asana*, the muscles of the back are stretched, the spinal column receives a rich supply of blood, and the thyroid gland is well massaged. Plow Pose prevents stiffening of the spine and obesity and removes various diseases of the liver, spleen, and stomach. It should be performed immediately after Shoulder Stand.

Method

1. Perform Shoulder Stand (Sarvanga Asana).

2. Keeping the legs straight and to-gether, exhale and bring the legs down and to the back until the toes touch the ground.

3. Keep the arms stretched along the ground and pointing away from the head and legs. Press the chest against the chin. Breathe normally as you hold the pose for as long as you can without straining.

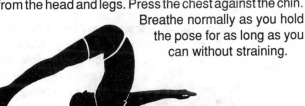

4. Slowly bring your legs down to the ground. Remain lying on your back and relax.

BRIDGE POSE

(Setubandha Asana)

This pose keeps the spine elastic and flexible. It is good to perform Bridge Pose immediately after Plow Pose since the spine is flexed in the opposite direction.

Method

1. Lying on your back, fold your legs, keeping the knees bent and feet flat on the floor.

2. With the elbows on the floor, arch the torso, supporting your back with the palms of your hands. Keep the head, neck and shoulders flat. Breathe normally and maintain the pose for as long as you can without feeling strain.

3. As a variation, you may then remove your hands from your back and grab your ankles, stretching your torso as much as possible. Again, breathe normally as you hold the pose.

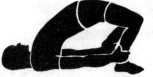

FISH POSE
(Matsya Asana)

Fish Pose prevents diseases of the stomach, lungs and throat. It renders the spine elastic, increases the capacity of the lungs, loosens the shoulder muscles, and increases the blood circulation throughout the body. Fish Pose also exercises the thyroid and parathyroid glands. It is a good compliment to the shoulder stand and plough poses and should be practised immediately following them.

**Method I
(Half Pose)**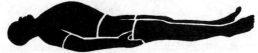

1. Lie on your back with your arms at your sides.
2. Pressing your elbows on the floor, arch your back and raise your chest and waist. Lift your chin and arch your neck backward as far as possible so that the top of the head rests on the floor. Since the chest is expanded to its fullest, breathe deeply through the nose.

**Method II
(Full Pose)**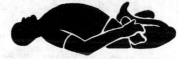

1. Assume Padma Asana (Lotus Pose): Sit with your legs stretched in front of you. Then, using your hands, place the right foot on the left thigh and the left foot on the right thigh. If Lotus Pose isn't possible for you, any cross-legged pose will do.
2. Keeping the legs crossed, lie on your back.
3. Supporting yourself by the elbows, raise your chest and waist off the ground. Arch your back and neck so that the top of the head rests on the floor. Grasp the toes with your fingers and hold. Since the chest is expanded to its fullest, breathe deeply through the nose.

COBRA POSE
(Bhujanga Asana)

"Bhujanga" means cobra. This pose is so-called because it resembles the raising of the cobra's hood. Cobra Pose increases the elasticity of the spine and, thereby, aids in the maintenance of overall sound health. It tones all the muscles of the back. It is especially useful for women in removing troubles of the reproductive organs. It removes constipation, regulates appetite and arouses kundalini energy.

Method

1. Relax face down on the ground, keeping the palms of the hands flat underneath the shoulders.

2. Inhale and raise the head, neck, and chest as a cobra raises its hood. Feel the stretch exerting an invigorating pressure down the spine from one vertebra to the next.

3. Continue to stretch backward while keeping the body from the navel to the toes in contact with the ground. Retain the breath as you hold the pose.

4. To return, exhale as you slowly lower yourself until the upper body is in the original prone position. Perform chin lock by pressing the chin gently into the chest.

LOCUST POSE
(Shalabha Asana)

Shalabha Asana resembles a locust with its tail up as it flies. This pose tones the abdominal muscles, liver, pancreas, and kidneys and removes various disorders associated with them.

It strengthens the lower back. Many troubles of the stomach are prevented through its regular practice. For best results, perform it immediately after Cobra Pose.

Method

1. Lie face down with the hands under the thighs, palms up. You may make a fist for better leverage.
2. Inhale as you stiffen the whole body, raising the legs as far as possible. The head is tilted back slightly so that the chin touches the ground. The body from the navel on up also remains touching the ground.
3. To return to prone position, slowly lower the legs while breathing out.

BOW POSE

(Dhanura Asana)

Combining the advantages of Cobra and Locust Pose, the Bow Pose offers a complete stretch along the whole length of the spine. It aids in relieving intestinal and digestive disorders. It normalizes appetite, reduces fat, and increases blood circulation in the abdominal region.

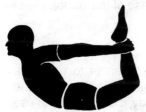

Method

1. Lie flat on your stomach. Fold your legs at the knees and bring your heels close to your bottom by grasping the ankles firmly.
2. Inhale as you raise the chest, shoulders, and knees by pulling the legs until your arched spine looks like an archer's bow and your arms its string. Retain the breath as you hold the pose and then exhale as you return to normal.

HEAD STAND
(Shirsha Asana)

The Head Stand pose endows one with fresh energy and luster. So numerous are its benefits to the body and mind that it is called the "king of all *asanas.*"

In daily life, the body is generally maintained in an erect position. In this position, certain valves within the veins continue to receive the same type of pressure. But when the body is reversed, the pressure points change. Now those valves that do not generally maintain pressure begin to do so, while the others begin to relax. This exerts a healthy and balancing influence on the whole physical system.

In Head Stand, the brain draws a rich supply of pure arterial blood. This is a boon to brain-workers since memory is improved and the nervous system is toned. A regular practitioner of this pose enjoys sound sleep. It helps cure varicose veins, removes defects of the liver, spleen, and lungs, and enhances the power of digestion.

Another powerful benefit of the Head Stand is that it aids in the transformation of sex energy into spiritual energy *(ojas shakti)*, thus helping one to practise meditation successfully.

Regular practice of Head Stand leads to natural *pranayama* (breath control) and the awakening of *kundalini shakti* (the mystic energy lying dormant at the base of the spine).

Method

1. Provide yourself with a folded blanket to use as a cushion for your head in this exercise. Since the top of the head will bear the full weight of the body, it is advisable to use the folded blanket to lessen this pressure.

2. Kneel down and with fingers interlocked rest the forearms on the cushion so they form two sides of a triangle.

2. Bend down now so that the top of the head rests on the cushion while the back of the head presses firmly against the

interlocked fingers to steady and support it.

3. Straighten the knees so that your body now forms an inverted "V," contacting the floor at only the forearms, head and toes.

4. Slowly walk towards your head, bringing your knees as close to the chest as possible. (Note: Practise up to this stage regularly for a month or until you feel confident enough to proceed further.)

5. Keeping your balance, continue the walking motion until the legs are automatically lifted. As they lift, keep the knees bent and thighs pressed against the chest, counterbalancing and preventing the body from falling forward.

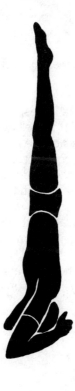

Now the body is inverted, supported on the head at the forearms. This phase of Shirsha Asana should be mastered before proceeding further.

In this phase, perfect balance and confidence is achieved without prematurely attempting the complete posture. Here the body is completely resting on the head in a straight line, yet the legs are still folded. The final stage is simply achieved:

6. Gently straighten the legs, keeping your balance by simultaneously straightening the knees and lifting the thighs. In this final pose, the legs and trunk of the body are in a straight line with the toes pointing upwards.

7. To return to your original position, slowly reverse the process described above.

8. It is important that after the practice of Shirsha Asana you lie down relaxed on your back until the blood circulation returns to normal.

HEAD-KNEE POSE
(Paschimottan Asana)

The Head-Knee Pose exercises many important muscles in the body and tones the nerves as well as the bladder and other internal organs. In addition, it helps to increase and maintain elasticity of the spine.

Method

1. Lie flat on your back with your arms stretched back over your head and resting on the floor.

2. Keep the legs fully extended with the knees locked as you inhale and slowly lift your upper body into sitting position.

3. Breathing out, stretch forward, catching your toes with your fingers.

4. In the final position, your head is between the knees, your legs are straight, and your arms are bent with the elbows resting on the floor. As you hold the pose, breathe normally. Hold the forward bent pose for a few seconds only. Repeat two to five times, according to your capacity.

5. Release the toes. Keeping the arms stretched up beside your head, inhale and come up, and then slowly lower yourself down into prone position.

WHEEL POSE
(Chakra Asana)

When this pose is perfected, the body resembles a wheel or *chakra*. It is one of the more rigorous of the backward bending exercises. All parts of the body—arms, chest, thighs, waist, and legs—are well exercised. One acquires perfect control of the body and an elastic spine which ensures a high standard of health, vitality, and agility. Wheel pose is an excellent compliment to Paschimottan Asana (Head-Knee Pose) since the spine is stretched in the opposite direction.

Method

1. Lie flat on your back.
2. Place your hands beside your head with the palms face down, the fingertips practically touching the shoulders and your elbows pointed up.
3. Bend your knees and keep the feet well-supported on the floor.
4. Inhaling, lift the body, keeping your weight on your hands and feet only.
5. According to your capacity, slowly move the feet closer to your hands to get the maximum stretch of the spine. As you hold the pose, retain the breath as long as possible and then continue to breathe normally. Feel a stream of *pranic* energy flowing from the base of the spine towards the brain.

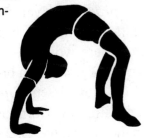

6. Exhale as you return to prone position.

PRANAYAMA EXERCISES

What is Prana?

Prana is the subtlest form of energy. As the universal storehouse of energy, it underlies all physical energies such as electricity, magnetism, light, heat, etc. and also sustains all mental processes such as thinking, feeling, willing, and reasoning. *Prana* is the manifestation of the Supreme Spirit as the sustainer of life and all forces in the world.

Due to *prana*, the ocean surges, the sun shines in the heavens, the stars move along their definite courses, and the earth and other planets revolve around the sun. Due to *prana*, the rivers flow towards the ocean and the mountains hold their heads high in the air. Without *prana*, there would be no life on earth. This is the meaning of *prana* in a broader sense.

In a limited sense, *prana* is the vital force that sustains life by performing various vital functions that keep the body alive. Breathing is one such such effect of *prana*. By controlling and harmonizing the breath, a yogi gains control over the subtle *prana*, which is linked to the mind and senses, which, in turn, are linked to the soul.

EXERCISES IN PRANAYAMA

Sukha Purvaka Pranayama

This *pranayama* is very effective in arousing the mystic powers of the spirit and is one of the most important exercises to practise every day. Such regular practise endows you with radiant health, a powerful memory, an abundance of energy, a magnetic personality, peace of mind, and purity of heart.

Sit comfortably, preferably in cross-legged position, with your spine straight. Using your right hand, place your thumb just to the side of your right nostril. Fold your index finger and middle finger to the palm and lightly place the fourth finger and pinky just to the side of your left nostril.

Close your right nostril with your thumb and inhale slowly through your left. This is called *purak* (inhalation). Next, close your left nostril with your fourth finger and pinky and, keeping both nostrils closed, hold the breath for as long as you can comfortably do so. This is *kumbhak* (retention). Then release the pressure of the thumb and exhale very slowly through your right nostril. This is called *rechak* (exhalation).

Repeat the exercise, this time inhaling through the right nostril and exhaling through the left, still keeping a comfortable period of retention in between. This constitutes one cycle of *Sukha Purvaka Pranayama*. Try to practise five of these cycles every day.

Kapala Bhati Pranayama

Regular practice of this exercise promotes purification of the lungs and the blood. It also tones the entire nervous system.

Sit comfortably, preferably in a cross-legged pose, with your spine straight. Exhale quickly and forcefully through the nose as you pull in the abdominal muscles sharply. Then relax those muscles, allowing air to flow into your lungs. Repeat this pattern of quick, vigorous exhalation followed by gentle inhalation ten times. Then inhale deeply, hold your breath as long as you can without discomfort, and exhale slowly. All the while, your mental attention should be focused on the exhalation process.

Bhastrika Pranayama

The term *"bhastrika"* means bellows and when this exercise is being practised, the breathing seems to imitate the rapid movement of a blacksmith's bellows. Regular practice of this *pranayama* gives warmth to the body and relieves asthma and inflammation of the nose and throat.

Exhale quickly and forcibly through the nose, pulling in the abdominal muscles, and then immediately inhale while relaxing the abdominal muscles. Repeat this ten times, making exhalation and inhalation follow each other rhythmically in rapid succession (like the panting of a dog). Then breathe in deeply, retain, and exhale slowly. Do this for three to four rounds. In this *pranayama* your mental attention is focused equally on exhalation and inhalation.

Shitali Pranayama

This is a cooling *pranayama* which quenches thirst and appeases hunger. Regular practice of this exercise purifies the blood and alleviates many physical problems. This *pranayama* should be practised after *Bhastrika Pranayama*.

Stick out your tongue and fold it lengthwise into a tube. Draw the air in through the folded tongue with a hissing sound. Then retain as long as you can without discomfort, keeping the mouth closed. Exhale slowly through both nostrils. This can be repeated six times.

Pranayama for Relaxation

Lie face up on the floor, on a bed, or on a reclining chair. Relax completely, from the toes to the head. Breathe in deeply and quietly and feel that you are filling yourself with energy, joy and peace. Then exhale slowly and comfortably, without even feeling aware that you are exhaling.

Mentally repeat "O...O..." while inhaling and "M...M..." while exhaling. *Om* is a symbol for God and repetition of this one-word *mantra* creates very positive and peaceful vibrations in the mind. You may also repeat any other *mantra*, half while inhaling, half while exhaling.

EXERCISES IN
BREATH AWARENESS
AND MEDITATION

• Breathe in an effortless, natural way and watch your breath. Feel that with each breath you are drawing cosmic energy from the ocean of universal life. This inhaled energy or *prana* is permeating every fiber of your being, every vein and artery, every nerve and cell of your body.

With each exhalation, feel that all the toxins from your body and all the complexes of your mind are being expelled. Gradually you are being attuned with the ocean of universal life.

• As you watch your normal breathing in an effortless way, feel your body absorbing energy through respiration. As the breath enters your lungs, feel that your body is like the ocean shore, receiving the tide upon its sandy beach. Like the beach, your body is exhilarated by the touch of the universal ocean of *prana*. Then with the outgoing breath, feel that the tide is turning back, leaving the sandy shore—and your body—refreshed. Your body is thus bathed and refreshed at every moment by the surging ocean of universal *prana*.

• While breathing in, feel that a stream of *OM*, permeated by the Divine Presence, is entering through your nostrils. With each incoming breath, feel that your consciousness is expanding gradually to infinity and that you are dissolving your ego in the vast expansion of the Self. With each outgoing breath, feel that you are gradually coming back from infinite expansion and returning to individual consciousness.

• Gently, without interference, observe your breathing and mentally associate the *SOHAM mantra* with your breath. Feel that the incoming breath represents *"SO,"* and the outgoing breath represents *"HAM."* *"SO"* means *"That"*—the Divine Self which is beyond the mind, senses, and ego. *"HAM"* means "I am." Thus, *SOHAM* means "That am I" and, with every breath you take, you are asserting your oneness with God, the Divine Self.

THE VALUE OF VEGETARIAN DIET

Pure food makes your body healthy and full of vitality, and helps keep your mind calm, balanced, and peaceful. Vegetarian food is purer than nonvegetarian food and, therefore, provides many benefits for body and mind. Furthermore, the human body is not well designed to receive nutrition from meat. Nutrition is assimilated more efficiently from a vegetarian diet.

Nonvegetarian food is risky for your health because so many artificial substances are given to commercially-raised animals. By eating meat, you are increasing the level of toxins in your body.

You also never know what diseases were present or about to develop in the animal's body when it was killed. These diseases may not be detected when the meat is inspected according to usual standards. There is a humorous anecdote about a man who was being served dinner at a party. When the meat was offered to him he declined, saying, "I will have everything else you have, but not the meat." "Why? Have you become a vegetarian?" the host asked. "Oh no," he replied. "I am a meat inspector and, therefore, I know the quality of that meat and where it came from!"

Being a vegetarian also helps you to maintain a more joyous and elevated state of mind. When you eat meat, one part of your mind knows how the animal was brought to the slaughter house and killed, how its entrails were removed, how it was cut up. However, one never wants to think about these things, especially while eating the meat.

Life is very dear to all animals. When an animal is killed, it experiences great fear, which is recorded in its body in a subtle way. So, when you later eat that animal, you are imbibing the impressions of that fright.

A carefully planned vegetarian diet, therefore, helps keep the body free of toxins and, most important of all, keeps the sensitive mind free of the subtle negative impressions that are generated by the killing of animals. If you are eating nonvegetarian food, you would benefit greatly by gradually moving away from it and beginning to enjoy more nourishing vegetarian food that can be prepared in the most delightful and flavorful ways.

THE SEARCH FOR BEAUTY

Amazing as it may seem, your body is not your real self! "You" are, in essence, a spirit, a soul. Your body is merely a vehicle that enables you to function in this world for the purpose of evolving spiritually and ultimately attaining Enlightenment or God-realization. As you grow up, your body changes in size, shape, strength, and health—and eventually dies. However, you are ever unchanging, imperishable, eternal. The real you is perfect.

When you were an infant, you were so tiny that an adult could just pick you up with one hand. Now your body has grown and changed considerably. Then and now, the inner you is the same. Even when death comes, you—as a spirit—will be the same. Like an old garment that gets thrown away and replaced, the body is discarded at the time of death and another one is acquired. But the real you has not been affected in any way.

If the body is not the real you at all, then why does the world give so much importance to it? Why are so many billions of dollars and billions of hours spent each year on beautifying the body and covering it with elegant clothing?

Like many people, you may feel that being beautiful pertains to one's physical appearance: having stylish clothes, a good-looking face, an attractive body. As you grow wiser, however, you will realize that real physical beauty depends on radiant health and abundant energy and that the highest form of beauty lies not in the body but in one's mind. You may, from an external point of view, be quite beautiful or handsome but internally you may be terribly burdened by ugly thoughts and feelings that disfigure your mind. Inner beautification is far more important than decorating what is on the surface.

The person who has devoted much time to caring for his external appearance, but has paid little attention to beautifying his mind, cultivates a beauty that is only "skin-deep." Profound beauty is "mind-deep"—it reflects a healthy and pure mind. The mind becomes a reservoir of beauty when it is filled with joyous thoughts, when it radiates harmony and peace, and when it is able to conquer anger with love, egoism with humility, and selfishness with generosity of the heart.

Yoga is a beautifying process that does not cost you anything. Furthermore, the results are permanent. All it requires is that you get up early in the morning, do some hatha yoga exercises, repeat *mantra* (a Divine name or a mystic formula), and practise meditation. Then with a relaxed mind, do your duties efficiently.

You will develop a sense of freedom and joyousness that will make you most beautiful.

When you are fulfilled, content, relaxed, and happy, a spiritual beauty manifests within you. This beauty is like the radiance and splendor of a magnificent tree in full bloom. It is not the artificial beauty that is worshipped by the world. In comparison to spiritual beauty, this artificial beauty is like paper flowers pasted on a paper tree to make it look as if it were blossoming!

It is important to take care of your body, but not to become obsessed by it. Don't waste all your time fussing over your looks, trying to decide whether putting one strand of hair over here and another over there makes you look more attractive. It is only when you begin to understand that you are not the body that your real beauty will manifest and you will become truly beautiful to everyone.

The Wrestler and the Beautiful Lady

Around the sixteenth century, there lived a young wrestler named Dhanurdas, who fell in love with a singer and soon married her.

Dhanurdas found his wife so beautiful that he could not take his eyes away from her. When they travelled during the hot Indian summer, he would hold an umbrella over her head and walk backwards so that he might keep her lovely face perpetually in view. Naturally, people laughed at such a spectacle but he didn't care what they thought. His wife, on the other hand, felt very uncomfortable about his behavior but, out of respect for the Hindu tradition, she had to accept whatever he did.

During one of their trips, a saintly person observed Dhanurdas' obsessive behavior and thought it very amusing; so he sent his disciples to fetch the infatuated wrestler. When the man came before him, the sage said, "I am very pleased that you are a lover of beauty."

"Thank you, most gracious sage," replied the young man. "My wife's beauty has so captivated my mind that I cannot take my eyes from her!"

"Because you admire beauty so much," the sage said, "I am going to conduct a special *puja* (worship) before the Deity and I want you to be present with me to receive God's blessings."

According to the story, the sage, by his spiritual power, transmitted to the young man a glimpse of God. As a result of that blessing, Dhanurdas was able to behold the infinite Divine beauty that pours through the universe like cascading waters, surging in the ocean, shining in the sun, shedding nectar through the moon, smiling through the radiant autumn forest.

The moment his mind captured a glimpse of that beauty, he was completely transformed. "Oh sage," said Dhanurdas, "hereafter God will be the object of my intense devotion. I shall not take my eyes from Him." He and his wife were then initiated as disciples and, in time, became highly advanced saints.

As this story shows, there is an extremely powerful urge in human personality to adore beauty. The fact is, however, that behind that urge is the search for God, Who is the embodiment of infinite beauty, and it is only in moving towards God that every aspect of your personality becomes beautiful.

The magic wand of Divine beauty is quite miraculous. Touched by that beauty, your intellect becomes reflective and increasingly more intuitive, the feelings of your heart begin to flow into the stream of Divine Love, your actions become selfless and increasingly more compassionate and magnanimous, and your mind becomes meditative, allowing you to enjoy serenity and inner peace.

Because beauty proceeds from God, it is "captured" in your personality just as the sun is captured in a clear lake. The more integrated and harmonized your personality becomes, the more you reflect the beauty of God and radiate its dazzling glory to others.

ENJOYING THE GIFT OF SLEEP

Healthy sleep is a great attainment. It is a sign of physical as well as psychological health. If your personality is highly integrated, you can control sleep and sleep at will.

Sleep is necessary so that the physical body can rest and recharge itself at the end of each day. During sleep, special physiological and chemical changes occur in the body. Your blood becomes more alkaline and nature works to expel toxins or poisons. Your tired body heals itself faster during sleep because your mind and ego do not interfere at that time.

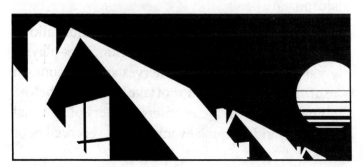

Sleep is a great aid in securing health, in promoting physical and mental balance, and in curing disease. In every way, it is a marvelous Divine medicine, given as a gift by nature.

Physical Hints for Promoting Healthy Sleep

- Do not depend on stimulants to keep awake or sleeping pills to go to sleep. Let sleep emerge naturally from your heart and bathe your body in fresh energy. The sleep produced under the influence of drugs is not as healing as natural sleep. These drugs depress your nerves, and your mind becomes duller and duller as time passes by.

- Practise hatha yoga's powerful exercises to promote flexibility and strength of the body, deep and complete breathing, and profound relaxation. These exercises recharge your physical body with *prana* (vital energy). As you continue doing them with regularity and precision, you will enjoy healthier sleep.

- Follow a sensible diet and eat in moderation, allowing adequate time for good digestion. Diet plays a great part in soothing your nerves and promoting a restful sleep. As a rule, do not take heavy food before going to sleep. In the *ashrams* (centers of spiritual learning) in India, the evening meal is served at or before sunset so that there is sufficient time for the food to be digested before the students go to sleep.

- Sleeping on your left side also helps to promote better sleep. This encourages the breath to flow through the right nostril, aiding in the assimilation and digestion of food, as well as providing other benefits to the body while it sleeps.

- Do not sleep with your head towards the north. To do so allows the polar magnetic pull to interfere with the functioning of your brain.

- A good principle to follow is, "Early to bed, early to rise." Set a definite time for going to sleep that utilizes your best energies and try to maintain it.

- Practise moderation in sleeping, eating, playing, studying, meditating, and in all aspects of your life. Too much or too little of anything can put stress on your nerves and disbalance your psychophysical personality.

Elevate Your Mind

Before going to sleep, try to elevate your mind. Read some elevating passages from an inspiring book, pray with a sincere heart, or repeat *mantra* (a Divine name or mystic formula) with feeling and devotion. The suggestions that you give to your mind before sleeping are carried to your unconscious in a spontaneous manner and they continue to operate during the night. Even if you read or pray for only five minutes, that effort educates your unconscious profoundly.

If you know the art of repeating *mantra* or the Divine name (such as Om, Sri Ram, Krishna, Jesus and others) with devotional feeling, you do not need any other form of lullaby. With each repetition, feel you are surrendering yourself to God, Who is the embodiment of love and sweetness. In this way, repetition of *mantra* gently rocks you to sleep, free of care and anxiety.

Repetition of the *mantra*, *Om Namo Narayanaya*, is a special yogic sleeping potion! According to Hindu mythology, the greatest sleeper in the world is God in the form of Lord Narayana, Who constantly sleeps on the couch of the Shesha serpent. In the twinkling of an eye, He creates the world and dissolves it but, unconcerned by all this, He continues to enjoy infinite peace and bliss. If you were to realize that Lord Narayana—the Divine Self—as the Reality within you, you too could experience the sleep of supreme peace at every moment.

You sleep most profoundly when your mind is awake to the higher Reality within, when you realize that your personality is a wave in the cosmic ocean of life, sustained with infinite compassion by Divine Will. When you discover that you do not carry the strings of your personality in your own hands but, rather, that you are ever in Divine Hands, you can easily allow your nerves to relax and carry you into deep, healthy sleep.

Keep Yourself Active

During the day, keep yourself active. Do not allow yourself to be *tamasic*, or filled with inertia. If you are confused about something and do not know what course of action to take, do not simply close your door, lie down on your bed, and remain morose and melancholy. Make every effort to resolve the situation and keep yourself active by practising *karma yoga* (selfless action). Tirelessly, use your talents and abilities for the good of others.

If you keep yourself active and useful to others, you will find that every obstruction in life will pass away. Fortified by the knowledge that the Self within you is bound to triumph, you will solve your problems effectively and be able to sleep profoundly and deeply.

Follow a Righteous Path

Live righteously so that you are not pinched by a guilty conscience. If you have done things that you should not have done, if you have hurt others and degraded yourself in your own eyes, your guilty conscience will rob you of your sleep by sending dark creatures of the unconscious winging their way into your dreams like vampires.

If you promote fraud, treachery, violence, and hatred, you cannot relax at bedtime and enjoy real rest. But, as you free yourself from grosser sentiments and integrate yourself in the light of yoga, you become able to relax your mind the moment you go to sleep and surrender serenely in Divine Hands.

The Supreme Commander
of Sleep

The yogic art of mastering sleep involves control of sleep in all its aspects. It involves allowing yourself, by your will, to flow into a peaceful sleep and transcend the conscious problems of life. It involves waking up with brightness and alertness. It involves being in command when sleep is trying to overpower you and you need to stay awake. It involves learning to take a quick "cat-nap" for a few minutes when your mind is drowsy but needs to be back on its feet quickly to continue working. It involves taking control of the entire process of sleeping and waking by your healthy will so that the demands of your life are handled with success and skill.

Therefore, learn the art of promoting sound and healthy physical sleep and learn to curb the dullness of mind that yogis refer to as psychological sleep. Most important of all, strive to attain God-realization, wherein you will discover what the sages mean by the "sleepless sleep of the Self." This is the sublime state of awareness enjoyed by the wise, the mystic sleep in which the world of day to day reality has faded from one's view and only the nondual Self remains!

GLOSSARY

Ahimsa: Nonviolence.

Akrodha: Absence of anger.

Apara Vidya: The relative knowledge that helps in daily life.

Aparigraha: Noncovetousness or nonhoarding of possessions you do not need.

Artha: Material value of life.

Asanas: Physical postures.

Ashram: Center of spiritual learning.

Ashramas: Stages in life.

Asteya: Nonstealing.

Atma Vinigraha: Control of mind.

Bhoga Buddhi: An intellect that is inclined only to sense-enjoyment.

Bhujanga Asana: Cobra pose.

Brahmacharya Ashrama: The student stage of life.

Brahmacharya: Vow of celibacy; a complete discipline of body, mind and senses.

Brahman: The Absolute, the Divine Self.

Chakra Asana: Wheel pose.

Dama: Control of senses.

Dhanura Asana: Bow pose.

Dharma Lakshanas: Characteristics of righteousness.

Dharma: Righteousness.

Dhee: Purity of intellect.

Dhriti: Firmness.

Gayatri Mantra: A vedic prayer for the enlightenment of intellect.

Gita: Srimad Bhagavad Gita, one of the most popular Hindu scriptures.

Grihastha Ashrama: Householder's stage of life.

Gunas: Modes of Nature: sattwa, rajas and tamas.

Guru: Spiritual preceptor, one who guides you on the path to Liberation.

Hala Asana: Plow pose.

Hatha Yoga: Branch of yoga consisting of asanas and pranayamas—psychophysical exercises.

Ishwar Pranidhan: Surrender to God.

Japa: Repetition of mantra.

Kama: Vital value of life.

Karmas: Actions performed by thought, word, and deed.

Kshama: Forgiveness, forbearance.

Kumbhak: Retention of breath.

Mahabharata: Hindu epic scripture.

Mala: Rosary of 108 beads.

Manasik: Mental repetition of mantra.

Mantra: A divine name or mystic formula.

Manu Smriti: A Hindu Scripture containing ethical laws.

Matsya Asana: Fish pose.

Mauna: The pratice of silence as austerity.

Moksha: Spiritual value of life, Liberation.

Naishthika Brahmachari: One who has taken the vow of brahmacharya for his whole life.

Nirvana: Liberation, the goal of life.

Niyamas: Ethical observances outlined in Raja Yoga.

Ojas Shakti: Spiritual energy.

Om: The sacred Name of God; the source of all mantras.

Pakoras, Rasgulas: Edible treats, sweets and savories popular in India.

Para Vidya: Mystical knowledge.

Paschimottan Asana: Head-knee pose.

Pranas: Vital forces.

Pranayamas: Breathing exercises.

Puja: Worship.

Purak: Inhalation of breath.

Rajas: Mental restlessness, distraction.

Ramayana: A Hindu scripture which tells the story of Rama.

Rechak: Exhalation of breath.

Sadachar: Good manners, the foundation for good education and true progress.

Sadhana: Spiritual discipline.

Samadhi: Mystic experience of superconsciousness.

Santosh: Contentment.

Sanyasa: Renunciation.

Sarvanga Asana: Shoulder stand.

Satsanga: Good association.

Sattwa: Mental purity, harmony.

Satyam or Satya: Truthfulness; Thinking, speaking and acting on the basis of truthfulness.

Setubandha Asana: Bridge pose.

Shalabha Asana: Locust pose.

Shaucha: Purity of body and mind.

Shirsha Asana: Head stand.

Shubha Samskaras: Pure impressions in the mind.

Surya Namaskar: Adorations to the Sun. Set of twelve poses in Hatha Yoga.

Swadhyaya: Study of scriptures and repetition of mantra.

Tamas: Mental dullness, negativity.

Tapas: Austerity.

Tattwas: Elements.

Tratak: Steady gazing with the eyes open.

Upanishads: Hindu Scriptures containing the wisdom of the Vedas

Upanshu: Semi-verbal repetition of Mantra.

Vaikhari: Loud repetition of mantra.

Vairagya: Dispassion.

Vanaprastha Ashrama: Retired stage of life.

Vedas: The four basic scriptures of the Hindus—Rik, Yaju, Sama and Atharva Vedas.

Vidya: Knowledge.

Viveka: Discrimination.

Yamas: Ethical restraints outlined in Raja Yoga.

About Swami Jyotirmayananda And His Ashram

Swami Jyotirmayananda was born on February 3, 1931, in a pious family in Dumari Buzurg, District Saran, Bihar, India—a northern province sanctified by the great Lord Buddha. From his early childhood he showed various marks of future saintliness. He was calm and reflective, compassionate to all, and a constant source of inspiration to all who came in contact with him. Side by side with his studies and practical duties, he reflected upon life's deeper purpose.

An overwhelming feeling to serve humanity through a spiritual life led him to embrace the ancient order of Sanyasa on February 3, 1953, at the age of 22. Living in the Himalayan retreats by the sacred River Ganges, he practised intense austerities. In tireless service of his Guru, Sri Swami Sivananda Maharaj, Swamiji taught at the Yoga Vedanta Forest Academy as a professor of religion. In addition to giving lectures on the Upanishads, Raja Yoga and all the important scriptures of India, he was the editor of the *Yoga Vedanta Journal*. Ever able to assist foreign students in their understanding of Yoga and Vedanta, his intuitive perception of their problems endeared him to all.

Swamiji's exemplary life, love towards all beings, great command of spiritual knowledge, and dynamic expositions on Yoga and Vedanta philosophy attracted enormous interest all over India. He frequently lectured by invitation at the All India Vedanta Conferences in Delhi, Amritsar, Ludhiana, and in other parts of India.

In 1962, after many requests, Swami Jyotirmayananda came to the West to spread the knowledge of India. As founder of Sanatan Dharma Mandir in Puerto Rico (1962-1969), Swamiji rendered unique service to humanity through his regular classes, weekly radio lectures in English and in Spanish, and numerous TV appearances.

In March, 1969, Swamiji moved to Miami, Florida, and established the ashram that has become the center for the international activities of the Yoga Research Foundation. Branches of this organization now exist throughout the world and spread the teachings of yoga to aspirants everywhere. In 1985, the Indian ashram near New Delhi opened its doors and is now serving the community by offering yoga classes, by publishing the Hindi Journal, *Yoganjali*, and by assisting the needy through a medical clinic.

Today Swami Jyotirmayananda occupies a place of the highest order among the international men of wisdom. He is well-recognized as the foremost proponent of Integral Yoga, a way of life and thought that synthesizes the various aspects of the ancient yoga tradition into a comprehensive plan of personality integration.

Through insightful lectures that bring inspiration to thousands who attend the conferences, camps and philosophical gatherings, Swamiji shares the range and richness of his knowledge of the great scriptures of the world.

His monthly magazine—*International Yoga Guide*—is enjoyed by spiritual seekers throughout the world. His numerous books and cassette tapes are enriching the lives of countless aspirants who have longed for spiritual guidance that makes the most profound secrets of yoga available to them in a manner that is joyous and practical.

Despite the international scope of his activities, Swamiji still maintains an intimate setting at his main ashram in Miami that allows fortunate aspirants to have the privilege of actually studying and working under his direct guidance. In the lecture hall of the Foundation, Swami Jyotirmayananda personally conducts an intense weekly schedule of classes in *Bhagavad Gita, Yoga Vasistha, Mahabharata, Upanishads, Panchadashi,* the *Bible*, Raja Yoga, Hatha Yoga and meditation.

With a work/study scholarship, qualified students are able to attend all classes conducted by Swamiji tuition-free. In return, students devote their energy and talents to the Foundation's noble mission by serving in the bookshop, offices, press, and computer and publication facilities.

Both the Yoga Research Foundation and the main ashram lie in the southwest section of Miami, two minutes from the University of Miami and 15 minutes from the Miami International Airport. The main ashram is on a two and a half acre plot surrounded by trees and exotic plants, reminiscent of the forest hermitages of the ancient sages. Adjoining are subsidiary ashrams that house student residents and Foundation guests. The grounds are picturesque, abounding with tall eucalyptus and oak trees, a fragrant mango orchard giving shelter to numerous birds and squirrels, and a lake of lotus blooms reflecting the expansion of the sky. In this serene yet dynamic environment, the holy presence of Swami Jyotirmayananda fills the atmosphere with the silent, powerful message of Truth, and the soul is nurtured and nourished, allowing for a total education and evolution of one's inner Self.

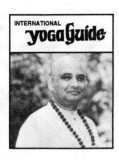

YOGA CAN CHANGE YOUR LIFE
Over 40 articles of practical guidance in applying Integral Yoga to your daily life.
paper: 240 pgs.   (Order No. 1) $4.99

CONCENTRATION AND MEDITATION
From beginning to advanced—a complete course in itself.
cloth: 200 pgs.   (2) $9.50

INTERNATIONAL YOGA GUIDE
12 monthly issues of the finest in Yoga teachings. (See Back Cover of this Catalog.)

YOGA GUIDE
Direct helpful answers to your questions on Yoga and life.
paper: 270 pgs.   (4) $2.99

THE MYSTERY OF THE SOUL (Katha Upanishad)
In story form, Katha Upanishad reveals its most profound teachings.
paper: 120 pgs.   (5) $2.99

THE WAY TO LIBERATION, Vols I & II
Yoga philosophy delightfully brought out through stories and dialogue from "Shanti Parva" of the Mahabharata—the well-known epic of India.
paper: 250 pgs.   (6a, 6b)   each $4.99

YOGA EXERCISES for Health and Happiness
Discover the key to a lifetime of health, beauty and profound peace of mind. Illustrated.
paper: 272 pgs.   (7) $4.99

DEATH AND REINCARNATION
Clarifies the mysteries of after-life, reincarnation and the Law of Karma.
cloth: 198 pgs.   (8) $9.50

RAJA YOGA—STUDY OF MIND
Detailed study allows the reader to experience and control the phenomenon of the mind.
cloth: 108 pgs.   (9) $9.50

MANTRA, KIRTANA, YANTRA AND TANTRA
Theory and practice of the simplest, most direct method to elevate the mind.
paper: 64 pgs.   (10) $3.99

HINDU GODS AND GODDESSES
Philosophy and mystic symbolism behind Hindu deities.
paper: 64 pgs.   (11) $3.99

BEAUTY AND HEALTH through Yoga Relaxation
Tap the boundless resources of the mind through the art of Yoga relaxation.
paper: 64 pgs.   (12) $1.99

YOGA QUOTATIONS
From the wisdom of Swami Jyotirmayananda, quotes for deep meditation and reflection.
paper: 240 pgs.   (13) $3.99

YOGA MYSTIC POEMS
Lofty verses reflecting the nature of the inner spirit.
paper: 240 pgs.   (14) $2.99

Books

YOGA MYSTIC SONGS for Meditation, Vols. I-VII
Spiritual music by Swami Lalitananda promoting a peaceful setting for meditation.
(15a-g)   each $2.99

YOGA IN LIFE
Practical essays by Swami Lalitananda for quick advancement in Yoga.
paper: 268 pgs.   (16) $2.99

YOGA MYSTIC STORIES
Insightful stories of great philosophical and mystic significance.
paper: 208 pgs.   (17) $3.99

YOGA STORIES AND PARABLES
Charming tales of great philosophical and mystic significance.
paper: 208 pgs.   (18) $3.99

RAJA YOGA SUTRAS
The original Sutras of Patanjali Maharshi with translation and in-depth commentary.
paper: 240 pgs.   (19) $2.99

YOGA WISDOM OF THE UPANISHAD
Classical exposition containing the essence of all Yoga philosophy.
paper: 240 pgs.   (20) $4.99

YOGA SECRETS OF PSYCHIC POWERS
Explore the mysterious powers of the mind in this fascinating manual.
paper: 208 pgs.   (21) $4.99

JNANA YOGA (Yoga Secrets of Wisdom)
Concise and comprehensive description of the Yoga of Knowledge.
paper: 64 pgs.   (22) $1.99

VEDANTA IN BRIEF
Acquire a knowledge of the basic structure of Vedanta philosophy in a very short time.
paper: 244 pgs.   (23) $3.99

YOGA VASISTHA, Vols. I, II & III
Rare account of Sage Vasistha's highest teachings to Lord Rama; the only exposition to be found in the West.
paper: 288 pgs. ea.   (24a, b, c)   each $4.99

SEX-SUBLIMATION, TRUTH & NON-VIOLENCE
Yoga explanation of basic ethical qualities universally adopted by all religions.
paper: 208 pgs.   (25) $3.99

APPLIED YOGA
Advanced application of Integral Yoga in your life.
cloth: 212 pgs.   (26) $9.50

YOGA OF PERFECTION (Srimad Bhagavad Gita)
The most loved and revered scripture in philosophical literature.
paper: 120 pgs.   (27) $3.99

WAKING, DREAM AND DEEP SLEEP
Unravels the puzzling nature of these three states of consciousness.
paper: 64 pgs.   (28) $2.99

Books

INTEGRAL YOGA—A Primer Course
Contains everything you need to get started on the road to a better life.
paper: 112 pgs. (29) $2.85

YOGA INTEGRAL—Curso Básico
Spanish translation of Integral Yoga—A Primer Course.
Paper: 112 pgs. (29S) $2.85

YOGA ESSAYS for Self-Improvement
Simple, practical and dynamic ways to life's enhancement.
paper: 248 pgs. (30) $4.99

THE YOGA OF DIVINE LOVE
A commentary on the Narada Bhakti Sutras.
paper: 240 pgs. (31) $4.99

INTEGRAL YOGA TODAY
Sunday afternoon talks at Miami's Theosophical Society.
paper: 96 pgs. (32) $2.50

YOGA OF ENLIGHTENMENT
Chapter 18 of the Bhagavad Gita—Sanskrit, translation and detailed commentary.
paper: 176 pgs. (33) $5.00

SRIMAD BHAGAVAD GITA
Pocket version with Sanskrit transliteration and English translation by Swami Jyotir-mayananda.
paper: 379 pgs. (34) $4.00

THE ART OF POSITIVE THINKING
Series of articles revealing the power of mind and the techniques used to unlock and cultivate this power.
paper: 145 pgs. (35) $3.50

EL ARTE DEL PENSAMIENTO POSITIVO
Spanish version of The Art of Positive Thinking.
paper: 160 pgs (35S) $3.50

THE MYSTICISM OF MOTHER WORSHIP
An inspiring and comprehensive exploration of the mysticism behind Devi Puja or Mother Worship.
paper: 70 pgs. (36) $10.00

ADVICE TO HOUSEHOLDERS
Insight into attaining the highest goal—Self-realization—while achieving harmony within the family unit, and between family and society.
paper: 174 pgs. (37) $4.95

ADVICE TO STUDENTS
Insight into the important questions facing young people as they strive to meet the challenges of life in today's world.
paper: 238 pgs. (38) $5.95

Cassettes

One-hour/$10.00 each

A number after a lecture topic in the following list indicates that there are other cassettes in the list which give insight into the same topic, although the lectures are not related sequentially. If you have difficulty finding any topic you are interested in, please write to us for help.

101
What Happens at the Time of Death
How to Overcome Loneliness #1

102
How to Cooperate with Others #1
How to Educate Your Children #1

103
Karma Yoga #1
How to Develop Vairagya (Dispassion) #1

104
How to Promote Cheerfulness #1
The Teachings of Lord Krishna

105
The Glory of Satsanga #1
How to Remember God #1

106
How to Develop Faith
How to Become a True Disciple #1

107
How to Develop Endurance #1
How to Develop Ahimsa (Nonviolence)

108
How to Develop Self-Confidence #1
How to Overcome Egoism #1

109
How to Remove Jealousy #1
How to Control Imagination #1

110
How to Overcome Dullness of Mind
How to Live in the Present

111
How to Develop the Art of Listening #1
How to Develop the Art of Speaking #1

112
How to Remove False Pride #1
The Practice of Yoga in the World

113
How to Remove Mental Abnormalities
How to Remove Mental Depression

114
What is True Religion? #1
What is God?

115
How to Study Scriptures
How to Be Magnanimous

116
How to Practice Kundalini Yoga #1
How to Develop Psychic Powers #1

117
Why a Yogi is a Vegetarian
Health in the Light of Yoga #1

118
How to Develop Your Talents
How to Utilize Your Time

119
How to Serve Humanity #1
How to Pray #1

120
How to Develop Discrimination #1
How to Practice Austerity

121
How to Think Positively
How to Promote Wisdom

122
How to be Truly Prosperous
How to Develop the Spirit of Service #2

123
How to Remove Ignorance
How to Develop Spiritual Aspiration

124
Spiritualism vs. Spirituality
How to Practice Meditation

125
How to Practice Truthfulness #1
What is Your Essential Nature

126
How to Withdraw the Senses
How to Educate the Subconscious

127
How to Develop Positive Imagination #2
How to Overcome Procrastination

128
How to Develop Inspiration
How to Overcome Maya

129
How to Cooperate with Others
All Pleasures are Painful to the Wise

130
How to Develop Foresight in Life
Fate and Free Will

131
How to Overcome Hatred #1
How to Enrich Your Life

132
How to Practice Relaxation #1
How to Acquire Spiritual Strength #1

133
How to Meditate on God
How to Practice Japa #1

134
How to Develop the Art of Adaptability #1
How to Promote True Culture

135
How to be Truly Awakened
Meditate on a Beautiful Scene of Nature

136
What Happens after Death
How to Prevent Crime in our Society

137
How to Promote Religious Unity
How to Develop Presence of Mind #1

138
How to Prevent Drug Addiction
Resolutions of the New Year #1

139
How to Practice Introspection
How to be Sincere

140
Overcome Destiny by Self-Effort #1
How to Control Desires #1

141
How to Integrate Your Personality
How to Control Desires #2

142
What is the Nature of the Soul
What is the Nature of the World-Process

143
What is Spiritual Evolution
How to Remember God #2

144
What is Dharma (Righteousness)
How to Face Adversity #1

145
How to Overcome Cowardliness
How to Develop Compassion

146
How to Remove Misunderstanding
How to Listen to the Voice of Conscience

147
How to Overcome Infatuation
How to Promote Mental Health #1

148
How to be an Ideal Disciple #2
How to Promote Unity of Man

149
How to Overcome Jealousy #2
How to Control Imagination #3

150
How to Solve Problems
How to Secure Goodwill of Others

151
How to Develop Presence of Mind #2
How to Develop Enthusiasm

152
Journey of Life
How You Can Change Your Life

153
The Message of the Gita
How to Elevate the Mind #1

154
How to Develop Promptness
How to be Rational

155
How to Draw Divine Grace
How to Develop Integrity

156
How to be Free from the Past #1
How to Overcome Pessimism

157
How to Overcome Gossiping
How to Live a Spiritual Life

158
Glory of Satsanga (Good-Association) #2
Practice of Vichar (Enquiry)

159
How to be an Effective Speaker #2
How to Develop Spiritual Strength #2

160
How to Practice Relaxation #2
How to be a Religious Person #2

161
What is the Law of Karma?
How to Develop Contentment

162
How to Face Adversity #2
How to Develop Cheerfulness #2

163
How to Promote Self-Analysis
Purpose of Life & Manner of Attaining It

164
How to Promote Universal Love
How to Overcome Self-Pity

165
The Art of Listening #2
The Art of Speaking #3

166
How to Develop Surrender to God #1
How to be a Karma Yogi

167
How to Overcome the Doubting Mind
Glory of Satsanga (Good-Association) #3

Cassettes

One-hour/$10.00 each

168
How to Remove Vanity #1
How to Elevate Your Mind #2

169
How to Practice Enquiry of 'Who Am I?' #1
How to Overcome Fear

170
How to Educate Your Children #2
How to Cooperate with Others #3

171
Parapsychology and Yoga
Yoga and Christianity #1

172
How to be Free from the Past #2
How to Practice Japa #2

173
Spiritual Resolves & How to Keep Them #2
How to Remove Anxiety #1

174
How to Develop Intuitional Knowledge
What is the Purpose of Suffering in Life?

175
How to Develop Psychic Powers #2
How to Practice Kundalini Yoga #2

176
How to Practice Truth #2
You are the Architect of Your Destiny #1

177
How to Pray #2
How to Serve Humanity #3

178
How to Develop Self-Confidence #2
Overcome Tendency to Commit Suicide

179
How to Overcome Craving
Overcome Destiny by Self Effort #2

180
Right Conduct and How to Promote It
How to Develop Endurance #2

181
How to Overcome Pride #2
Kriya Yoga

182
How to Practice Integral Yoga
How to Practice Vairagya (Dispassion) #2

183
The Art of Reflection
How to Develop Endurance #3

184
Yoga and Christianity #2
Judaism in the Light of Yoga

185
How to Overcome Greed
How to Practice Adaptability #2

186
Simple Living and High Thinking #1
How to Promote Thought Power

187
Goal of Life
How to Realize 'Inaction' in Action

188
How to Develop Spirit of Renunciation
How to Remove Mental Conflicts

189
Progress and How to Promote It
You are the Architect of Your Destiny #2

190
How to Develop Surrender to God #2
How to Overcome Laziness

191
How to Overcome Mental Stress
Insight into Yoga Ethics

192
How to Enhance Health and Vitality #2
How to Develop Mental Health #2

193
How to be a True Sadhaka (Aspirant)
How to Overcome Anxiety #2

194
How to Overcome Vanity #2
How to Develop Equal Vision

195
How to Practice Moderation
Enquiry of 'Who Am I?' #2

196
How to See the Positive in Others
Simple Living and High Thinking #2

197
Karma Yoga #2
Raja Yoga

198
Bhakti Yoga
Jnana Yoga

199
How to Attain Mental Serenity
How to Practice Vairagya (Dispassion) #3

200
How to Attain Cosmic Consciousness
How to Practice Self-Discipline

201
The Art of Being Selfless
How to Pray #3

202
How to Experience Bliss
How to Overcome Intolerance

203
Parables in Spiritual Teachings
Characteristics of Spiritual Progress

204
How to Overcome Hatred #2
Resolutions of a Yogi #3

205
Tantra Yoga
Recreation

206
How to be Free of Bondage
The Significance of Tat Twam Asi

207
How to Overcome Tamas
How to Overcome Rajas

208
How to Promote Sattwa
Charity

209
How to Overcome Stress #2
How to Enjoy Peace

210
How to Practice Discrimination #2
How to Overcome Loneliness #2

211
Necessity of Guru
How to Be Free From The Past #3

212
How to Serve Humanity #3
How to Develop Compassion #2

601
Select Meditation Tapes (over 300)

602
Hatha Yoga Exercises

603
Concentration and Meditation

604
What is Yoga?

605
You are the Architect of Your Destiny

606
How to Acquire Peace of Mind

607
How to Remove Pain

608
The Story of Rama

609
Life and Teachings of Guru Nanak

610
Mind in Yoga Philosophy

611
Yoga Relaxation Exercises

612
Yoga Mystic Songs for Meditation

613
Raja Yoga: Two Lesson Course

614
The Control of Mind

615
The Path of Love

616
Where is Happiness?

617
Who Am I?

618
How to Solve Problems

Cassettes

One-hour/$10.00 each

701
Dispassion
Discrimination
Mental Serenity

702
Control of Senses
Faith
Endurance

703
Mental Tranquility
Renunciation of Selfish Actions
Aspiration for Self-Realization

704
Listening
Reflection
Vedantic Meditation

705
Nonviolence
Truth
Sex-Restraint

706
Nonstealing
Noncovetousness
How to Overcome Fear

707
As the New Year Begins
Mental and Physical Purity
Contentment
Austerity

708
Study of Scriptures
Repetition of Mantra
Surrender to God
Attitude Towards Others I

709
Attitude Towards Others II
Building of Character
Fearlessness
Purity of Nature

710
Steadiness In Wisdom
Charity
Renunciation
Absence of Fault-Finding Nature

711
Compassion
Absence of Greed
Absence of Fickleness
Forbearance

712
Humility
Hypocrisy
Arrogance
Pride

713
Good Association
Serenity
Enquiry
Contentment

714
Concentration
Meditation
Samadhi (Superconsciousness)
Repetition of Mantra

715
Intro to Upasana (Devout Meditation)
Om Upasana
Dahara Upasana
Shandilya Upasana

716
Madhu Vidya Upasana
Madhu Vidya Upasana
Antarayami Upasana
Samvarga Upasana

717
Prana Upasana I
Prana Upasana II
Bhuma Upasana
Soham Upasana

718
Akshara Vidya Upasana
Vibhuti Yoga Upasana
Gayatri Upasana
Maha Mrityunjaya Upasana

719
Kundalini Upasana I
Kundalini Upasana II
Kundalini Upasana III
Kundalini Upasana IV

720
Kundalini Upasana V (Muladhara)
Kundalini Upasana VI (Swadhishthana)
Kundalini Upasana VII (Manipura)
Kundalini Upasana VIII (Anahata)

721
Kundalini Upasana IX (Vishuddhi)
Kundalini Upasana X (Ajna)
Kundalini Upasana XI (Sahasrara)
Saguna Upasana I

722
Saguna Upasana II
Saguna Upasana III
Vichar (Enquiry) I
Vichar (Enquiry) II

723
Vichar (Enquiry) III
Vichar (Enquiry) IV
Vichar (Enquiry) V
How to Brighten the Intellect

Cassettes

One-hour/$10.00 each

724
Practice of Austerity
Karma Yoga I
Karma Yoga II
Karma Yoga III

725
Controlling the Mind
Surrender to God
Self-Discipline
Mystic Art of Prayer I

726
Mystic Art of Prayer II
Mystic Art of Prayer III
Your Essential Nature
Secret of Sadhana (Spiritual Discipline)

727
Positive Thinking I
Positive Thinking II
Positive Thinking III
Positive Thinking IV

728
Positive Thinking V
Positive Thinking VI
Positive Thinking VII
Positive Thinking VIII

729
Spiritual Value of Conflict
Secret of Yoga
Perseverance
Power of Mind

730
Bhavana I (Spiritual Feeling)
Bhavana II
Bhavana III
Bhavana IV

731
Bhavana V
Bhavana VI
Bhavana VII
Bhavana VIII

732
Evil of Procrastination
Spiritual Value of Life
Spiritual Lessons I
Spiritual Lessons II

733
Overcome Maya I
Overcome Maya II
Overcome Maya III
Overcome Maya IV

734
Overcome Maya V
What is Success?
What is True Education?
Glory of Satsanga (Good Association)

735
Selfless Service I
Selfless Service II
Selfless Service III
Develop Sattwa (Purity)

736
Remembrance of God
Self-Effort and Divine Grace I
Self-Effort and Divine Grace II
Secrets of Success

737
Experience of Enlightenment
Remove Mental Stress I
Remove Mental Stress II
Practice of Detachment

VIDEO TAPES

S-1	Positive Thinking, Vedanta in Practice, Guru Purnima Message.	$45.00
S-2	Satsanga with Swamiji, Insight into Dharma, Law of Karma.	$45.00
S-3	Birthday Message 1987, Christmas Message, Talk on Austerity.	$45.00
H-1	Hatha Yoga	$35.00

Cassettes

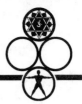

One-hour/$10.00 each

800
Art of Self-Discipline
Secret of Renunciation

801
Secret of Self-Restraint
Insight into Faith

802
Overcome Worry I
Overcome Worry II

803
Overcome Worry III
Practice of Reflection

804
Acquire Contentment
Spiritual Transformation

805
Reflection on Brahman I
Reflection on Brahman II

806
Power of Devotion
Remembrance of God

807
Glory of Divine Name I
Glory of Divine Name II

808
Illusion of the World-Process
Tat Twam Asi—THOU ART THAT

809
Insight into Nonduality
Path of Nivritti (Renunciation)

810
The Secret of Freedom
How to be Unshaken by Adversity

811
Disease of the World-Process
Your Spiritual Identity

812
How to Attain Peace
Mystic Art of God-Realization

813
How to Develop Divine Virtues
Insight into Ego

814
Insight into Intuition
Insight into Bhakti (Devotion)

815
Overcoming Insecurity in Life I
Overcoming Insecurity in Life II

816
Secrets of Success
Prevent Mental Abnormalities

817
Five States of Mind I
Five States of Mind II

818
Five States of Mind III
Five States of Mind IV

819
Five States of Mind V
Insight into Sadhana (Spiritual Discipline)

820
Insight into the Kleshas (Afflictions)
Insight into Vrittis I (Thought-Waves)

821
Insight into Vrittis II
Insight into Vrittis III

822
Insight into Austerity I
Insight into Austerity II

823
Swadhyaya (Study of Scriptures)
Surrender to God

824
Health and Physical Diseases
Mental Diseases

825
Overcoming Inertia
Overcoming Doubt

826
Overcoming Obstacles
Dream and Deep Sleep

827
Glory of Divine Name I
Glory of Divine Name II

828
Developing Dispassion
Overcoming Pessimism

829
Yogic Skill in Action
Essentials for Self-Realization

830
Qualities of a Karma Yogi
Equal Vision

831
Insight into Willpower I
Insight into Willpower II

832
Insight into Willpower III
Overcome Stress

833
Thought Culture I
Thought Culture II

834
Insight into Sleep I
Insight into Sleep II

835
Dream I
Dream II

836
Insight into Religion
Law of Karma

837
Vedanta in Practice
Quest for Love

838
Insight into Dharma (Righteousness)
Rise and Fall of Ego

839
Who Am I? I
Who Am I? II

840
Who Am I? III
Who Am I? IV

841
Three States of Consciousness I
Three States of Consciousness II

842
Three States of Consciousness III
How to Develop Purity of Intellect

843
Destruction of Vasanas (Subtle Desires)
Insight into Knowledge of Truth

844
Insight into Bondage and Release
Reason and Intuition

845
Quest for Happiness I
Quest for Happiness II

846
Quest for Happiness III
Quest for Happiness IV

847
Philosophy of Action I
Philosophy of Action II

848
Practice of Meditation I
Practice of Meditation II

849
Practice of Meditation III
Art of Relaxing the Mind

850
Insight into Freedom
Insight into Upasana (Devout Meditation)

851
Insight into Spiritual Progress
Insight into Self-Effort

852
Insight into Knowledge
Insight into Nonduality

853
Insight into Energy
Prophecy vs. Spirituality

854
Insight into Happiness
How to Overcome Mental Stress

855
How to Develop Cheerfulness
The Virtue of Self-Reliance

856
What Is Religion?
Insight into Hinduism

857
The Story of Prahlad
The Story of Druva

858
Message of Divali
The Destruction of Kamsa

859
What is True Education
The Mysticism of Devi Puja

860
Insight into Devotion
Instructions for Developing Devotion

861
Insight into Education
Success in Sadhana

862
Insight into Spiritual Aspiration
Removing Body Idea

863
How to Develop Devotion to God
Your Spiritual Identity

864
Insight into Sadhana (Spiritual Discipline)
Philosophy of Beauty

865
Insight into Peace
Potentiality of the Soul

866
Power of Devotion (Story of Sage Ambarish)
Insight into Nonviolence

867
Art of Handling Adversity
Be Practical

868
Divine Incarnation
Presence of God

869
Insight into Spirituality
Yoga in Practice

870
Insight into Grace
The Problem of Sin

871
Overcoming Intolerance
The Spiritual Path

Cassettes

45-minute/$5.00 each

872
Insight into Self-Effort
Insight into Memory

873
How to Develop Pure Intellect
How to Promote Sattwa

874
The Virtue of Perseverance
Insight into Optimism

875
The Virtue of Vigilance
Insight into Prosperity

876
The Practice of Humility
Insight into Integrity

877
Insight into Inspiration
The Art of Moderation

878
Insight into Swadhyaya (Study of Scriptures)
Overcome the Worrying Habit

880
The Value of Patience
The Virtue of Cheerfulness

881
Don't Look Back
The Philosophy of Desires

882
The Philosophy of Expectations
Prayer

883
Insight into Knowledge
Always be Thoughtful

884
How to Conserve Mental Energy
Insight into Good Manners

885
How to Overcome Insecurity
Insight into Sadhana (Spiritual Discipline)

886
Insight into Abhyasa (Repeated Effort)
Insight into Vairagya (Dispassion)

887
How to Handle Grief
How to Overcome Demoniac Qualities

888
Insight into Bliss
The Philosophy of Time

889
Insight into Bhavana (Devotional Feeling)
How to Overcome Hatred

890
How to Overcome the Sense of Insecurity
The Virtue of Patience

891
How to Overcome Prejudice
Insight into Selfless Action

892
Insight into Worship
Insight into Prosperity

893
A Message for Students
Insight into Death

894
How to Overcome Mental Distraction
Insight into Dharma

895
Insight into Compassion
Insight into Faith

896
Insight into Foresight
How to Develop Fortitude

897
Develop Purity of Intellect
The Philosophy of War

898
The Evils of Revenge
Insight into Egoism

899
Mysticism of Shivaratri
Overcoming Intolerance

900
Insight into Liberation
The Virtue of Patience

901
Insight into Renunciation
The Philosophy of Idol Worship

902
The Virtue of Fortitude
Imagination

903
Fate and Free Will
The Quest for Peace

904
Insight into Death
Insight into Miracles

905
How to Face Adversity
Insight into Detachment

906
Purity of Intellect
Tenacity

907
Insight into Nonduality
Insight into Dharma (Righteousness)

908
Insight into Meditation I
Insight into Meditation II

BOOKS: See book list on pages 242—244 for the order number and current price of each book.

CASSETTES: See cassette list on pages 245—253. Cassettes in the 100-700 series are 60 minutes long—$10 each. Cassettes in the 800 series are 45 minutes long—$5 each. Write us also about cassette series on various scriptures such as: *Gita, Upanishads, Bible, Ramayana, Yoga Vasistha, Mahabharata*, etc.

MAGAZINE: INTERNATIONAL YOGA GUIDE—$15/12 monthly issues; $27/2 years; $38/3 yrs; $12/year for more than 3 years; $300/lifetime subscription. Domestic postage prepaid. Foreign postage, per year: Canada $10.00, Mexico $8.25, All other countries $11.25.

This sheet may be torn out of the book and used as an order form, or it may be photocopied. Or you may simply send us the information in a letter. Be sure, however, to include all information asked for, especially the information on any credit cards used.

ORDER FORM

Telephone Orders: Call (305) 666-2006. Have your VISA or MasterCard ready.

Postal Orders: Please fill out the following information and send to the Yoga Research Foundation, 6111 S.W. 74th Avenue, South Miami, Florida 33143, U.S.A.

Please send the following books or cassettes. I understand that I may return any item for a full refund, or cancel my subscription to the *International Yoga Guide* magazine for a prorated refund.

QTY	ORDER NO. / TITLE	EACH	PRICE
*MEMBERSHIP: When you subscribe to the *International Yoga Guide*, you are automatically a member of the Yoga Research Foundation. All standing member/subscribers are entitled to 1) A 10% discount on all cassette and book orders, 2) 50% off all IYG back issues, and 3) Personal correspondence with Swami Jyotirmayananda on any question or difficulty.	SUBTOTAL	
		DISCOUNT*	
		SUBTOTAL	
		POSTAGE	
		TOTAL	

Sales Tax: For orders being sent to Florida, please add 6% to your order.

Shipping: 1st item $1.00 (U.S.) or $1.50 (foreign). Add each additional item: $.50 (U.S.) or $.75 (foreign). For magazine postage, see other side.

Name: _____

Address: _____

City: _____ State:_____ Zip:_____

Payment: Please send payment with your order. U.S. customers pay by money order or check payable to the Yoga Research Foundation, or credit card (VISA or MasterCard). Foreign customers pay in U.S. dollars by an international money order or check drawn on a U.S. bank. Please, no cash. All prices subject to change.

Credit Card Orders: VISA or MasterCard:

Card Number:_____ Expiration Date:____/____

Name on Card: _____

Signature: _____